Roland Hetzer (Ed.) ■ **Lung Transplantation**

Roland Hetzer

Editor

Lung Transplantation

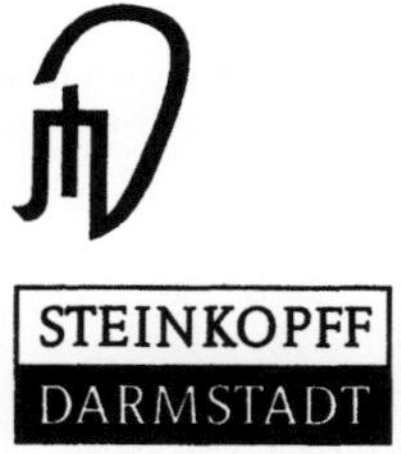

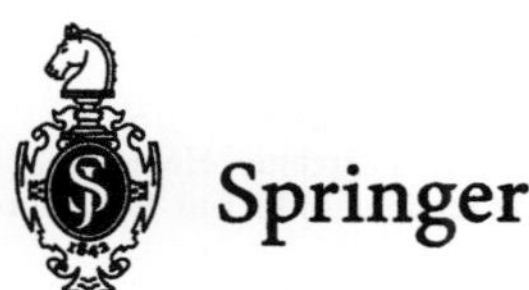

Springer

Roland Hetzer, M.D.
German Heart Institute Berlin
Augustenburger Platz 1
13353 Berlin, Germany

ISBN 978-3-662-04679-1   ISBN 978-3-662-04677-7 (eBook)
DOI 10.1007/978-3-662-04677-7

Cataloging-in-Publication Data applied for
Bibliographic information published by Die Deutsche Bibliothek. Die Deutsche Bibliothek lists this publication in
the Deutsche Nationalbibliografie; detailed bibliographic data is available in the Internet at http://dnb.ddb.de

http://www.steinkopff.springer.de
© Springer-Verlag Berlin Heidelberg 2003
Originally published by Steinkopff Verlag Darmstadt in 2003.
Softcover reprint of the hardcover 1st edition 2003

Production: Heinz J. Schäfer
Cover Design: Erich Kirchner, Heidelberg
Typesetting: Macmillan India Ltd. Bangalore

SPIN 10536176   85/7231 – 5 4 3 2 1 0 – Printed on acid-free paper

Preface

Clinical lung transplantation has seen an early start within the history of solid organ transplantation, marked by the 1963 first lung transplant by James D. Hardy. This was prompted by the seemingly easy way of joining the transplanted organ to the recipient by means of a few well-defined anastomoses, i.e. bronchus, pulmonary artery and pulmonary vein carrying left atrial cuff.

The following decade thus witnessed a number of such mostly unilateral lung transplants in several centres, in Germany represented by the two only lung transplants performed by E. S. Bücherl, then at the Neukölln City Hospital in Berlin in 1969. As with most other such attempts these two patients suffered early and lethal graft failure. There was only one single lung transplant patient who lived up to ten months after the transplant at Gent, Belgium, having been operated on by Derom in 1969.

The almost universal failure during this initial phase was attributed to bronchial anastomotic insufficiency, pulmonary infection of either the transplanted lung or the left-in-place contralateral lung and a far-reaching lack of knowledge how to cope with transplant rejection. In the early 1970s it had become generally accepted that lung transplantation could not be performed successfully.

Credit must be given to Bruce Reitz of Stanford for having resurrected lung transplantation by systematic and thorough experimental preparation and a very successful consecutive clinical series of combined heart and lung transplantation in 1981. Combined heart and lung transplantation in fact had been attempted by pioneers as Cooley and Barnard in the early 1970s, however, without success.

Following Reitz's stimulating achievement, pulmonary surgeons at Toronto, in particular Joel Cooper, started to tackle the seemingly insurmountable obstacles to isolated lung transplantation which then has been rewarded by astoundingly good results since 1982. Hence, lung transplantation has seen widespread clinical application and a vast number of experimental studies in order to ameliorate the fate of patients with otherwise untreatable diseases of the pulmonary parenchyma and the pulmonary vessels.

Much knowledge and experience has been accumulated since which, however, has not yielded the good results of other organ transplant endeavours, such as with kidney, liver and heart so far. More than in patients with such organ transplants the course after lung transplant has been afflicted with specific complications, i.e. infection, bronchial anastomotic complications and with the menacing transplant disease "bronchial obliterative syndrome" (BOS) which has remains to be the final and up to now more or less untractable curse in many of the transplanted patients.

The specific causes of the unsatisfactory situation are the exposure of the transplanted organ to the germ-laden outside environment, the weak spot of bronchial blood supply at the anastomoses, the difficulty in differentiating between infection and rejection and the inability to successfully treat BOS, to name only the most significant.

Still, some important revelations and changes of concept have been achieved, such as the recognition of cystic fibrosis being a very favorable condition for lung transplant in spite of the fact of chronic overgrowth of the bronchial tree with malignant bacteria. Furthermore, the technical requirements for good bronchial anastomosis and healing have been recognized and interventional bronchoscopy with its modern time armatorium of take-down of granulations, bronchial dilatation, and stent implantation has greatly helped to deal with bronchial sequelae. There has been some progress in recognizing rejection from endobronchial biopsy or from open lung biopsy material and the question of bronchial artery revascularization has been discussed repeatedly.

Heart and lung transplantation has now been reserved by most units to the end-stage complex congenital heart disease patients and bilateral lung transplantation has become the preferred procedure for the majority of diseases. There also have been some attempts to transplant pulmonary lobes in case of small recipient pleural cavity and in children, in this case also applying the concept of living-donor organ sharing.

At the Deutsches Herzzentrum Berlin pulmonary transplantation started in 1987 with three cases of combined heart and lung transplant, however, with only short-term success. Further preparations were made and in 1990 unilateral and bilateral lung transplantation was restarted, then with results comparable to those of other units that treat larger patient series. By now 79 combined heart- and lung transplants and 177 mostly bilateral lung transplants have been performed at this institution.

In 1996 a symposium with an international lineup of guests, including some of the most eminent experts in the field, was held in Berlin.

The proceedings of the symposium were planned and announced to be published in a symposium book. Many of the contributors sent us their manuscripts, some did not, and I am sorry to say that among the latter were some outstanding world authorities. After many requests to obtain the complete array of manuscripts and after repeated update of those authors complying with our pledge we decided to publish the booklet as it is after it has been waiting on my desk for several months.

Now the proceedings volume will be issued, representing the state of lung transplant specialists' thoughts and experiences of the period between 1996 and 2001. Not too much further progress has been made since and most of the articles are quite valuable to today's specialists.

I would like to express my thanks to the patient contributors to this volume who by now must have lost hope to see their articles printed and to Mrs. Ibkendanz and Dr. Gasser of Steinkopff Verlag for their continuing effort to finish this work. Finally my gratitude goes to the "Gesellschaft der Freunde des Deutschen Herzzentrums Berlin e.V." for their generous contribution to the editing and printing costs of this book.

Berlin, August 2002   Roland Hetzer

Contents

Single versus bilateral lung transplantation

H. C. Doerge, G. Wieselthaler, A. Zuckermann, O. Artemiou, O. Senbaklavaci,
W. Klepetko

Department of Thoracic and Cardiovascular Surgery, University of Vienna, Vienna,
Austria

Introduction

Following the initial success with heart/lung transplantation in Stanford (8), the first
successful single lung transplant was accomplished by the Toronto team in 1983 (9). In
recent years phenomenal progress has been made in the application of lung transplantation for patients with end-stage pulmonary disease. Experiences of individual
groups have challenged old dogmas and led to new approaches in all facets of lung
transplantation. However, it still remains in debate which form of lung transplantation represents the optimal treatment for the specific indications. Despite the clinical
acceptance of both, single and double lung transplantation, their role and potential
has still to be determined. This refers to the clarification of the ideal indications, to the
functional benefit, as well as to the long-term outcome that can be reached with each
technique. In this chapter, the various aspects of single and double lung transplantation are discussed.

Technique

The surgical techniques employed in single-lung transplantation (SLT) have not
changed substantially over the ensuing years and are now well established. Pneumec-
tomy is performed via a standard posterolateral thoracotomy. With the aid of
single-lung ventilation cardiopulmonary bypass support will not be required in most
transplantations. In cases of inadequate oxygenation and hemodynamic instability,
cardiopulmonary bypass can be employed by using the femoral vessels or, on the
right side, the right atrium and ascending aorta for cannulation. The bronchial
anastomosis is carried out in a simply end-to-end technique, using sutures on the
membraneous portion and single stitches on the cartilagineous portion. Alternatively,
the telescope-technique can be applied to construct the bronchial anastomosis. An
atrial cuff is built up by joining the superior and inferior veins to perform the venous
anastomosis. The arterial end-to-end anastomosis is constructed using a running
suture.

The incidence of bronchial anastomosis complications, a major problem in the past,
has decreased significantly. The occurence of bronchial dehiscence and/or stenosis is
now quoted to be 5 to 8% of cases (1). However, most bronchial complications are not
related to technical mistakes, but represent the sequellae of airway ischemia. The basic

principles in avoiding these complications are the preparation of a short donor bronchus with preservation of peribronchial tissue. Most centers have abandoned the technique of wrapping the bronchus with omentum or a vascularized intercostal muscle bundle since no beneficial effect on the prevention of bronchial dehiscence and/or stenosis has been documented (6). Bronchial revascularization by means of the internal thoracic artery or by direct implantation of bronchial arteries in the aorta is currently performed in only a few centers (2, 3).

It was previously thought that bilateral lung replacement required combined heart-lung transplantation. Subsequently, preservation of the recipient's heart was enabled by developing the en bloc double-lung technique. However, the technical complexity of the en bloc procedure, the necessity to use cardiopulmonary bypass and cardioplegic arrest and, moreover, the high incidence of donor airway ischemic complications associated with it led to the development of a bilateral sequential lung transplantation technique (BLT). An anterior bilateral thoracosternotomy (clamshell-incision) is employed which permits adequate exposure for safe excision and implantation of both lungs in sequence. The avoidance of cardiopulmonary bypass is possible in most cases, if the side with the least function is transplanted first. The sequential transplantation of each side is performed in an identical way as in single-lung transplantation.

Both techniques, SLT and BLT, are today well established and routinely performed in many centers with only minor variations. Although BLT is a substantially more expanded procedure than SLT, no difference regarding perioperative mortality has been documented in the International Registry (4).

General considerations

There are several main issues to be considered in choosing the appropriate transplantation procedure for a given patient and indication. Generally, the operation affording the highest degree of operative safety has to be offered in any instance. The determination of whether this is SLT or BLT must be tailored to the individual patient. Besides the point of safety, the operation that is likely to provide the greatest cardiopulmonary rehabilitation should be chosen. These decisions must be made taking into consideration the patient's acuity of illness and prognosis for short-time survival. The indications for 149 lung transplantions, 77 SLT and 72 BLT, at the University of Vienna are shown in Fig. 1.

SLT provides several potential advantages over bilateral lung replacement. Foremost is the prospect of increasing the number of transplants by performing two single transplantations rather than one bilateral transplantation. Moreover, SLT is a technically easier and shorter procedure that rarely requires cardiopulmonary bypass. SLT also allows the use of one lung from donors whose contralateral lung is injured or otherwise unsuitable for transplantation. On the other hand, BLT provides maximal functional improvement and, in contrast to SLT, much more respiratory reserve.

Over the last decade, the single-lung procedure has found application in the treatment of a variety of end-stage lung disorders, including restrictive and obstructive lung diseases and hypertensive pulmonary vascular diseases. There is no discussion regarding the role of SLT in patients with fibrosis, just as it is generally accepted that the appropriate treatment in patients with infectious pulmonary disease

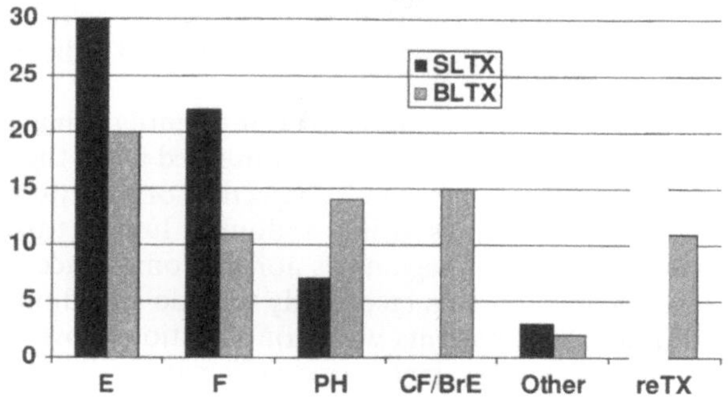

Fig. 1. Transplants by diagnosis. 149 lung transplantations (77 SLT; 72 BLT), University of Vienna 11/89–2/96. E: emphysema; F: pulmonary fibrosis; PH: pulmonary hypertension; CF/BrE: cystic fibrosis/bronchiectasis; reTX: retransplantation

is bilateral lung replacement. Although it has been demonstrated clinically that SLT is feasible in obstructive pulmonary diseases and pulmonary vascular disease, it still remains in debate whether it really represents the optimal form of treatment for these patients.

Indications

Fibrosis

Initial experience proved that pulmonary fibrosis was particularly suited to single lung replacement because the low lung compliance and increased vascular resistance of the native lung would ensure preferential ventilation and perfusion to the transplanted lung. Furthermore, the oversizing effect of the transplanted lung with regard to the usually small thoracic volume in patients with restrictive pulmonary disease provides a maximal benefit in lung function. The procedure can be performed without cardiopulmonary bypass in most cases.

In contrast to the common problems resulting with reperfusion edema after SLT in patients with primary pulmonary disease, as discussed below, this complication seldom occurs in patients with pulmonary fibrosis, even if their pulmonary pressure is significantly elevated. This is due to the considerably lesser extent of hypertrophy of the right ventricle in recipients with restrictive lung disease compared to those with primary pulmonary hypertension.

Obstructive lung diseases

Much of the early experience with SLT in recipients with obstructive lung diseases implied that this approach was associated with hyperinflation of the remaining native lung, causing secondary mediastinal shifting and ventilation-perfusion imbalance. Concern about this problem led to speculation that bilateral lung replacement would be necessary in all patients with obstructive lung diseases. However, subsequently the feasibility and efficacy of SLT has been confirmed in these patients, and until now emphysema has become the most common indication for successful transplantation of a single lung (4).

Temporary problems concerning ventilation imbalance with mediastinal shifting to the transplanted lung are only observed when the compliance of the transplanted lung is impaired either by severe rejection or infection. In this situation, separate ventilation of both lungs using a double lumen tube can become necessary until the transplanted lung regains its normal compliance (Fig. 2a, b). However, these problems can usually be managed easily and do not diminish the value of SLT as preferred treatment for patients with non-infectious obstructive lung diseases.

Selection of patients, especially patients with obstructive lung diseases, for SLT implies freedom from recurrent respiratory infectious episodes. Therefore every effort must be made during preoperative patient work-up to preclude the remaining lung from acting as a potential source for bacterial or fungal infections. In individual cases where this cannot be proven, a strong argument exists to prefer BLT to SLT.

Pulmonary hypertension

Clinical experience proved that SLT can effectively reduce even severely elevated pulmonary vascular resistance, resulting in dramatic improvement of right ventricular function (7). However, this also implies that the majority of cardiac output is immediately directed to the transplanted lung which, at this time, is more or less

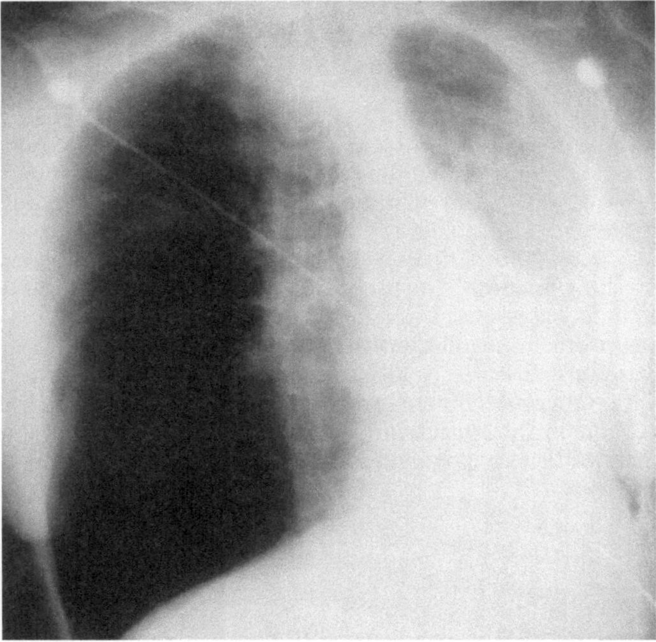

(a)

Fig. 2. a) Acute rejection on the 7th post-operative day after SLT for emphysema. After reinturbation of the patient, marked mediastinal shifting due to hyperinflation of the native lung has occurred. **b)** Intubation with a double lumen tube and separate ventilation normalizes the position of the mediastinum again and allows the transplanted lung to re-expand

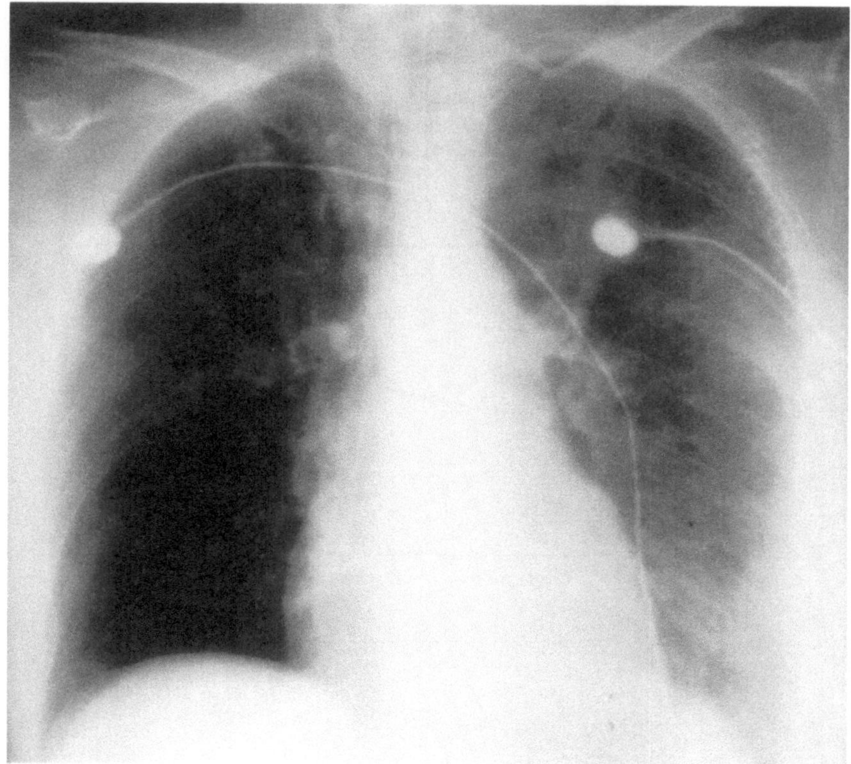

(b)

Fig. 2. Continued

compromised by the ischemic storage. As a consequence, frequent problems in the early postoperative period are reperfusion edema and remarkable hemodynamic instability, making the postoperative treatment of these patients especially demanding.

Beside these problems in the immediate postoperative period, late function of single-lung grafts in patients with pulmonary hypertension can be significantly compromised, whenever problems like infection, bronchial stenosis or chronic rejection occur. In these clinical situations, ventilation is shifted back to the native lung, whereas perfusion still preferentially passes the transplanted lung, which can lead to a marked ventilation-perfusion mismatch.

To overcome these problems, we have abandoned the concept of SLT for treatment of pulmonary hypertension and now regard BLT as the procedure of choice for this indication.

Late results

Looking at late results after lung transplantation, there has not been a significant difference documented in actuarial survival regarding the two procedures. This is true as well as in overall survival for all indications as in survival differentiated by indication (4).

Quality of life after SLT compared to BLT remains a point of ongoing discussion. In Fig. 3 the values of FEVI, pO2 and 6-min walk test in 20 patients (10 SLT; 10 BLT) with obstructive lung diseases transplanted at our institution are illustrated. As one would expect, FEVI reaches 50–60% of predicted values after SLT, in contrast to

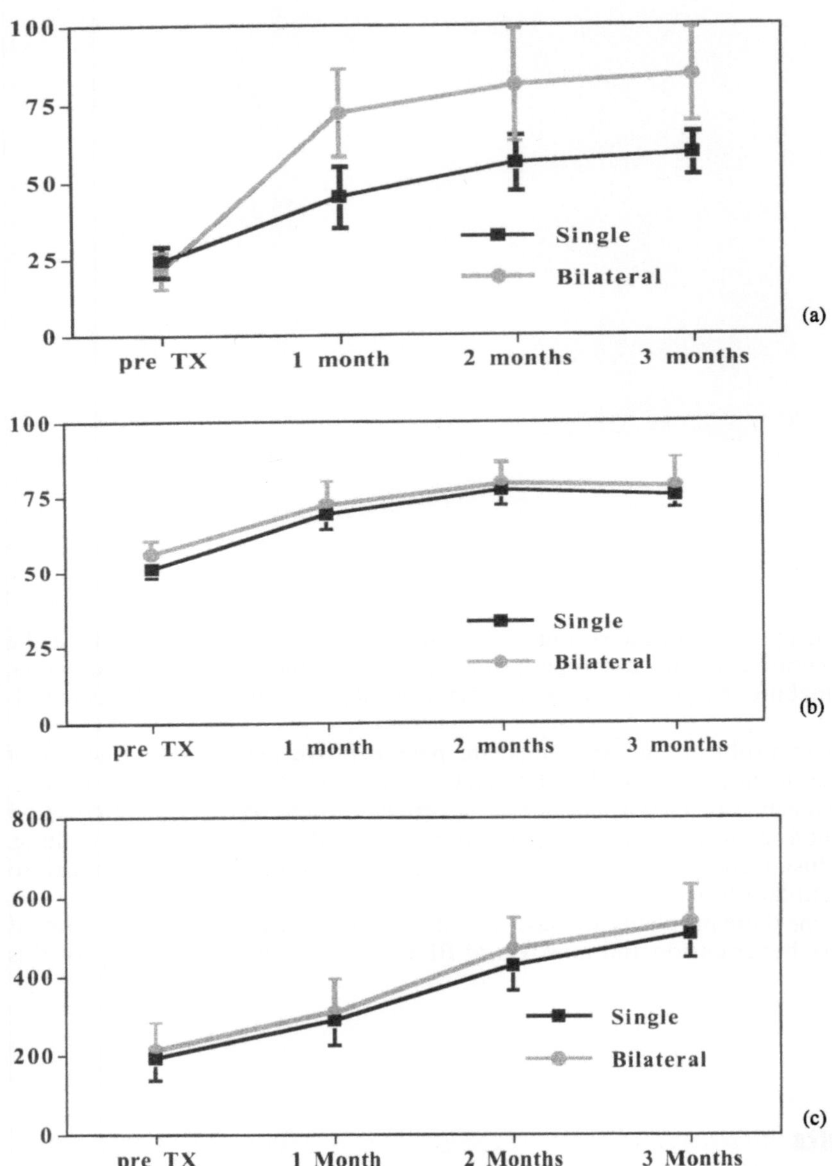

Fig. 3. Functional results of 20 patients with emphysema under going lung transplantation (10 SLT; 10 BLT). **a)** FEVI: percent predicted ($P < 0.005$); **b)** pO2: mmHG (n.s.); **c)** 6-min walk: meters (n.s.)

80–90% after BLT. That this does not necessarily result in better exercise tolerance of the BLT group is an important finding in view of the question of whether BLT should be offered routinely to young patients [5]. In recent papers it has been demonstrated that the improvement or near normalization of lung function is not necessarily followed by a normalization of exercise capacity and maximum oxygen up take [10]. Similar results have been described after combined HLT. This gives evidence that improvements in maximal work capacity can be reached only by regular aerobic training. It therefore seems reasonable to restrict BLT only to the group of patients who are capable and willing to undergo such a program. In contrast, the amount of improvement in lung function can become important as a functional reserve at a time of chronic graft rejection and obliterative bronchiolitis. Patients after BLT do remarkably better in this situation when compared to patients after SLT. This is true especially for the subgroup in which the course of chronic rejection can be stabilized with augmented immunosuppression at a somewhat lower level of pulmonary function. At present, the importance of this functional reserve of the BLT patient compared to the SLT patient has not yet been determined completely.

Conclusions

SLT remains the procedure of choice for patients with idiopathic pulmonary fibrosis and other interstitial lung diseases (e.g., lymphangioleiomyomatosis, lymphocytic interstitial pneumonitis). SLT also offers excellent therapy for patients with obstructive airways diseases. BLT is the procedure of choice for patients with infectious diseases (e.g., cystic fibrosis, bronchiectasis). In the interest of increasing the safety of the operation and the perioperative period it appears that BLT is indicated in the treatment of pulmonary hypertension. However, despite the wide experience with SLT and BLT, the particular value of both procedures remains still in discussion, and the debate regarding the most appropriate transplant procedure continues.

References

1. Cooper JD, Patterson GA, Trulock EP et al. (1994) Results of single and bilateral lung transplantation in 131 consecutive recipients. J Thorac Cardiovasc Surg 107: 460–471.
2. Couraud L, Martigne C, Velly J et al. (1992) Bronchial revascularisation in double-lung transplantation: A series of eight patients. Ann Thorac Surg 53: 88–94.
3. Daly RC, Tadjkarinai S, Khaghani A, Banner NR, Yacoub MH (1993) Successful double-lung transplantation with direct bronchial revascularization. Ann Thorac Surg 56: 885–892.
4. Hosenpud JD, Novick RJ, Breen TJ, Keck B, Daily P (1995) The Registry of the International Society for Heart and Lung Transplantation: Twelth official report-1995. J He Lung Transplant 14: 805–815.
5. Low DE, Trulock EP, Kaiser LR, Pasque MK, Dresler C, Ettinger N, Cooper JD (1992) Morbidity, mortality, and early results of single versus bilateral lung transplantation for emphysema. J Thorac Cardiovasc Surg 103: 1119–1126.
6. Miller JD, de Hoyos A, Patterson GA (1993) An evaluation of the role of omentopexy and early postoperative corticosteroids in clinical lung transplantation. J Thorac Cardiovasc Surg 105: 247–252.
7. Pasque MK, Trulock EP, Kaiser LR, Cooper JD (1991) Single lung transplantation for pulmonary hypertension: three month hemodynamic follow-up. Circulation 84(6): 2275–2279.

8. Reitz BA, Wallwork JL, Hunt SA, Pennock JL, Billingham ME, Oyer PE, Stinson EB, Shumway NE (1982) Heart-lung transplantation: Successful therapy for patients with pulmonary vascular disease. N Engl J Med 306: 557–564.
9. The Toronto Lung Transplant Group (1986) Unilateral lung transplantation for pulmonary fibrosis. N Engl J Med 314: 1140–1145.
10. Williams TJ, Patterson GA, Zamel N, Maurer JR (1992) Maximal exercise testing in single and double lung transplant recipients. Am Rev Respir Dis 145: 101–105.

Authors' address:
Walter Klepetko, M.D.
Department of Thoracic and Cardiovascular Surgery
University of Vienna, AKH Wien
Währinger Gürtel 18-20
1090 Wien, Austria

Rejection and infection after lung transplantation

M. Hummel

German Heart Institute Berlin, Berlin

Rejection

Introduction

Aside from early graft failure, surgical-technical problems and bronchial anastomotic complications, rejection and infection are the most important determinants of early and intermediate outcome after heart-lung and lung transplantation. Rejection of the solid organ allograft lung is a cell-mediated immunologic process initiated by the recognition of foreign MHC class II antigens. Acute rejection is predominantly a T-lymphocyte-mediated phenomenon. However, humoral immunity also plays a role in this process. Histopathologically, acute rejection is characterized by both perivascular mononuclear infiltrates and a lymphocytic bronchitis and/or bronchiolitis. Approximately all recipients of lung allografts experience clinical episodes of acute rejection and have histopathological correlates (1). A working formulation for classification and grading of pulmonary rejection has been proposed by the Lung Rejection Study Group of the International Society for Heart and Lung Transplantation for uniform reporting of histological evidence of lung allograft rejection (2).

Mechanisms of rejection

Lung allografts are transplanted along with a large complement of immunocompetent cells comprised of alveolar and airway macrophages and lymphocytes, hilar and pulmonary lymph nodes, and the bronchus-associated lymphoid tissue known as BALT. The bronchus-associated lymphoid tissue (BALT) seems to play an important role in the rejection process of the lung allograft (3, 4, 5). The BALT is part of the reticuloendothelial system and incorporated in the physiological recirculation pathway of lymphocytes. Analysis of HLA markers on cells recovered by bronchoalveolar lavage (BAL) indicates that rapid replacement of donor lymphocytes and macrophages occurs, such that the vast majority of BAL lymphocytes and macrophages are of recipient origin by 90 days after transplantation.

After transplantation, recipient recirculating lymphocytes continue along these physiological pathways, even in allograft lungs, so that BALT is the prime site of early infiltration by recipient lymphocytes (Fig 1). Upon arrival to the allograft's BALT, recipients respond against the graft's lymphocytes and other BALT cells provoking an *in situ* mixed lymphocyte reaction. At the end of the vascular rejection phase, large areas of BALT are occupied by immunoblasts (Fig 2). Finally, dissemination of activated lymphocytes from the BALT into the lymphoid tissues of the recipient consisting of the lung-associated lymph nodes (LALN), the spleen and the bone

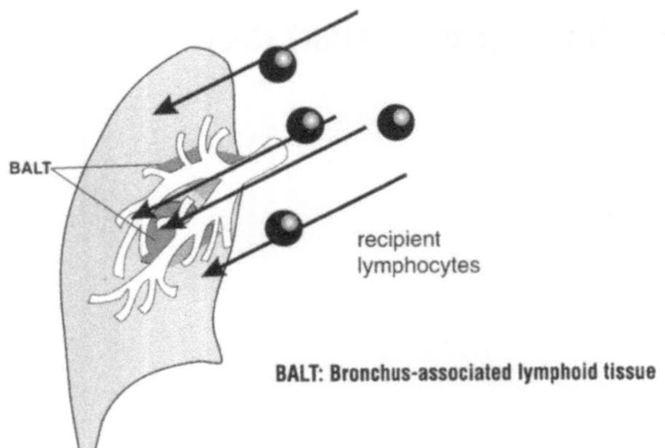

Fig. 1. Infiltration by recipient lymphocytes into the bronchus-associated lymphoid tissue. Adapted from: Prop J et al. Lung allograft rejection in the rat II. Transplantation 1985;40:126-131

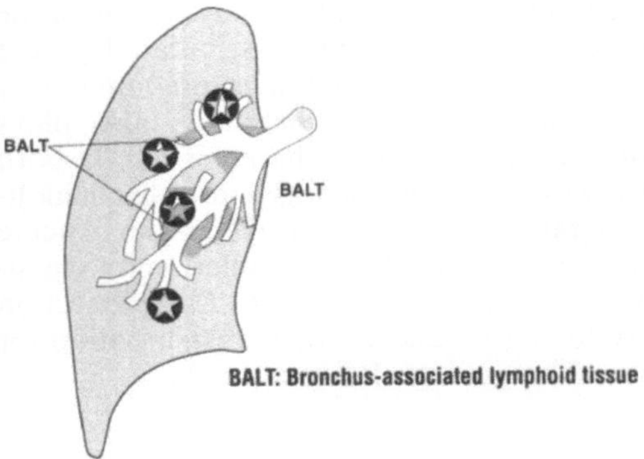

Fig. 2. Immediate direct stimulation of the infiltrating recipient lymphocytes in the bronchus-associated tissue. Adapted from: Prop J et al. Lung allograft rejection in the rat II. Transplantation 1985;40:126-131

marrow, results in a systemic stimulation of rejection (Fig 3). This passively transferred bronchus associated lymphoid tissue might explain why lung allografts are more vigorously rejected than other transplanted organs (6). Therefore, it is not surprising that the majority of lung transplant recipients experience at least one episode of acute rejection during the first 3 post-transplant months and that the lung allograft is much more likely to undergo acute rejection than is the cardiac allograft in heart-lung recipients. Furthermore, and in contrast to other transplanted solid organs, significant expression of MHC classes I and II antigens can be detected on tracheal, bronchial epithelium and vascular endothelium regardless of the rejection or infection status of the lung allograft.

Prophylactic immunosuppression

To prevent acute lung allograft, we use triple drug immunosuppression with preoperative loading doses of azathioprine (5 mg/kg bw orally) and cyclosporine

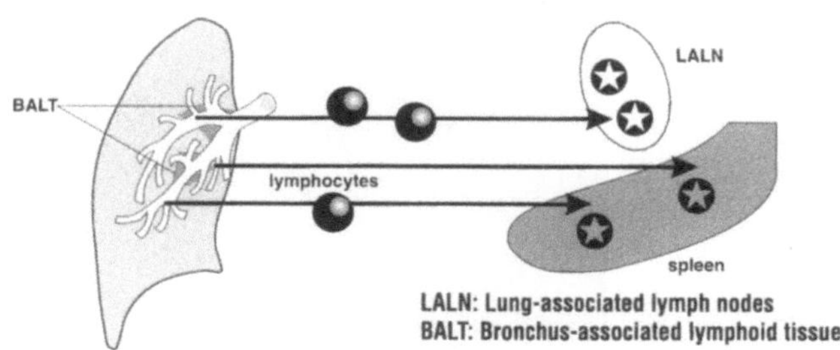

Fig. 3. Dissemination of lymphocytes from bronchus-associated tissue into lymphoid tissue of the recipient. Adapted from: Prop J et al. Lung allograft rejection in the rat II. Transplantation 1985;40:126-131

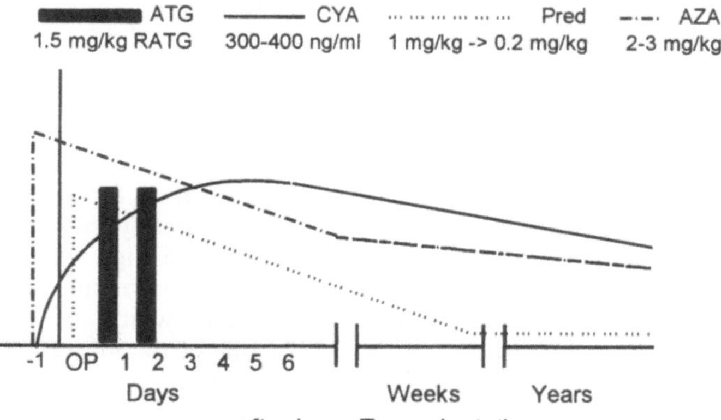

Fig. 4. Immunosuppression after lung transplantation

(4 mg/kg bw orally), intraoperative single dose methylprednisolone (1 g) and postoperative high dose steroids of 125 mg methylprednisolone every 8 h four times together with a short course of rabbit antilymphocyte globulin. Steroids are tapered within 60 days from 1 mg/kg bw to 0.2 mg/kg bw. Cyclosporine is given in divided doses b.i.d. and in children or patients with cystic fibrosis t.i.d. either orally or in cases of initial poor absorption intravenously. Azathioprine is maintained at 2–3 mg/kg/day orally or rarely intravenously while monitoring hematologic and hepatic parameters. To avoid infectious complications, in particular CMV- and EBV-reactivation and disease, prophylactic cytolytic induction therapy with ATG is restricted to a short time period of 1 or 2 days until cyclosporine trough levels, determined by monoclonal antibodies, are up to about 250–350 ng/ml which means unspecific cyclosporine levels of about 1000 to 1200 ng/ml. Later, if the patient can tolerate it, we try to bring whole-blood cyclosporine trough levels up to 400 ng/ml (monoclonal antibodies) or higher for about 3 months (Fig. 4).

To reduce the risk of acute renal failure induced by acute cyclosporine nephrotoxicity and prophylactic antibiotic therapy, Urodilatin, the human renal natriuretic

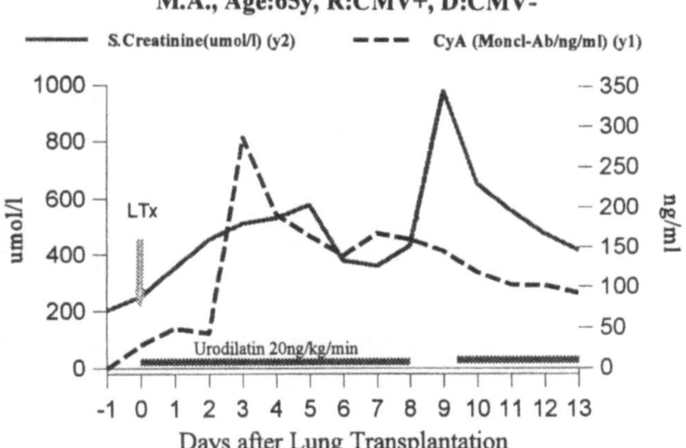

Fig. 5. Course of cyclosporine A trough levels and serumcreatinine over 13 days after double lung transplantation in a patient with prophylactic administration of Urodilatin (20 ng/kg/min). Rapid increase of serumcreatinine after stopping Urodilatin infusion on day 8. Drop of seumcreatinine after reinstitution of Urodilatin application during the next 4 days

peptide, which is an analogue to the circulating hANF, is administered immediately after transplantation by a continuous infusion of 20-40 ng/kg/min for about 4–8 days (Fig 5). The prophylactic application of this renal peptide, already shown to be beneficial after heart transplantation, enables early postoperative high whole-blood levels of cyclosporine in most patients without major renal impairment, thus avoiding the necessity of prolonged application of cytolytic agents which are the major risk factors for CMV-replication, disease, and probably one of the important determinants of the development of obliterative bronchiolitis and lymphoproliferative disease (7).

Acute rejection episodes

Acute rejection episodes which may occur as early as 5–7 days after lung transplantation, mostly accompanied by unspecific clinical symptoms like malaise, low-grade fever, dyspnea and/or cough, and deterioration of pulmonary gas exchange often associated with radiological signs of pleural effusion, mildly increased bilateral interstitial pattern or frank infiltrates are treated with boluses of 0.5 g methylprednisolone for 3 days after infections are ruled out essentially by rapid assessment for infectious causes with bacteriological and mycological examinations of sputum or bronchoalveolar lavage (BAL). Transbronchial biopsy at this stage is rarely helpful, since there are often diffuse non-specific histological findings. If the etiologies of these findings are correctly diagnosed as rejection, most if not all of the changes will have improved or resolved within 8–12 h following. A worsening picture leads to aggressive search for less obvious infectious causes, problems with the vascular anastomoses or a more severe rejection which may be refractory to steroids.

Both open-lung and transbronchial biopsies (TBB) have been used for histological examination of acute pulmonary rejection. Although there is a working formulation and a precise description for the grading of acute lung rejection, it is often difficult to make a differential diagnosis between rejection and infection solely on histologic examination of lung biopsy. For example, perivascular infiltrates, and peribronchial inflammation, which were initially believed to be specific for pulmonary rejection occur as well in about 50% of pulmonary CMV infection (8). Additionally, and in contrast to heart transplantation, rejection and CMV infection may coexist in the tissue.

Controversies in the diagnosis of acute lung rejection

Because of these difficulties and the necessity of other diagnostic approaches there are controversies in the diagnosis of lung rejection:

- What is the role of transbronchial biopsy?
- What is the role of noninvasive rejection diagnosis?
- How specific are the morphologic changes of acute cellular rejection (ACR) and obliterative bronchiolitis (OB)?
- How do biopsy grade and treatment choices correspond?

Role of transbronchial biopsy: The ability of transbronchial biopsy to act as a useful tool is dependent on the skill of the bronchoscopist and pathologist, the ability to obtain adequate samples, and the number of parenchymal fragments obtained. For acute rejection, greater than five and up to 15 parenchymal biopsies will lead to accurate diagnosis of rejection in more than 90% of cases (2, 9, 10). The same is true for documenting pulmonary infection. Whether transbronchial biopsy is useful in diagnosing obliterative bronchiolitis is questionable (11).

Lavage is excellent at documenting infection, however, it is not as specific as transbronchial biopsy. Compared to the importance for the diagnosis of infection, BAL is of little value because of a poor sensitivity in the detection of acute lung rejection (18).

Role of noninvasive rejection diagnosis: Pulmonary function measurements have shown to be important methods for early detection of acute lung rejection. The most predictive value reflecting deterioration of the small airway dynamics during acute rejection was reduction of FEV1 and FEF 25-75 (19, 20), which can be determined easily and daily by use of home spirometry. The validity of the procedure, however, depends on an acceptable baseline whereby each patient serves as his or her own control (Fig. 6). Compared to spirometries in patients with acute lung rejection, infection was not associated with significant deterioration of FEV1 and FEF 25-75, but did cause a significant fall in PaO2 (Fig. 7) (19). In the first postoperative month chest radiographs are abnormal in nearly all patients experiencing rejection or infection. In biopsy-proven rejection changes are often associated with pleural effusions, ill-defined nodules and mildly increased bilateral interstitial pattern. However, these changes are not specific and can also be seen with CMV pneumonitis. After the second posttransplantation month, chest radiographs are frequently normal even in case of acute rejection (21).

To present, no single immunological parameter is known to allow adequate monitoring of acute pulmonary rejection. Although IL-2 and IL-2R serum levels are elevated during acute rejection episodes, overlapping of serum concentrations in patients with rejection and infection does not allow accurate diagnosis. IL-2R levels are not specific for any one disease process but reflect the state of T-cell activation (22).

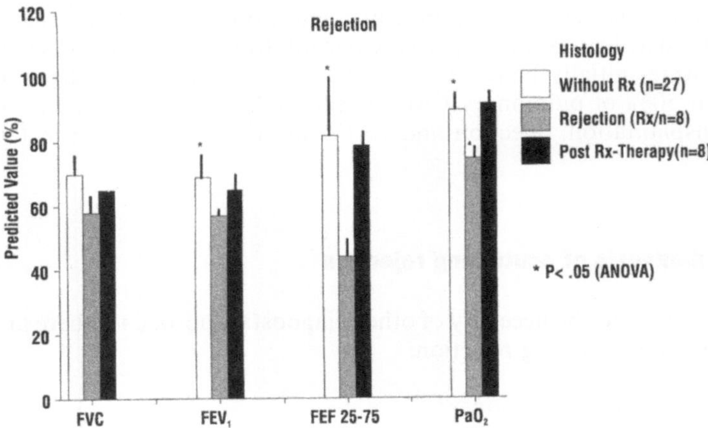

Fig. 6. Pulmonary function studies after lung transplantation - Rejection. Adapted from: Starnes VA et al. J Thorac Cardiovasc Surg 1989;98:683-690

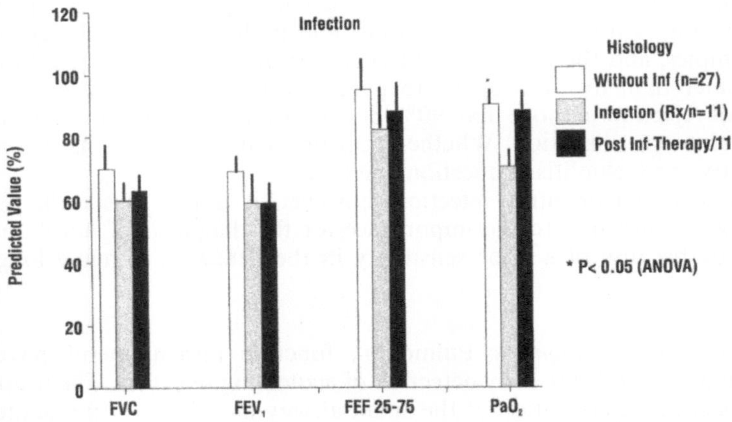

Fig. 7. Pulmonary function studies after lung transplantation - Infection. Adapted from: Starnes VA et al. J Thorac Cardiovasc Surg 1989;98:683-690

Specificity of morphologic changes of acute cellular rejection (ACR) and obliterative bronchiolitis (OB): The presence of perivascular mononuclear cell infiltrates is not specific for acute cellular rejection (ACR) because some infections like cytomegalovirus (CMV) pneumonitis and even chronic *Pseudomonas* and *Staphylococcus* colonization and infection may cause similar histological features in about 20–50% of cases (8, 12). On the other hand, fibrous tissue in transbronchial biopsies as a sensitive marker of bronchiolar obliteration can be detected with high accuracy in transbronchial biopsies (13), but only 40% of these patients have developed obliterative bronchiolitis within 2 years of follow-up (9, 14).

Correlation between biopsy grade and choice of treatment: As in heart transplantation, correlation between the histological grade of acute rejection and the severity of symptoms or function test abnormalities is not very good. From a immunophenotypical perspective, acute cellular rejection is dominated by helper T-cells with a small number of B-cells (15). HLA class II antigens are expressed to a greater level on endothelium and epithelium (16, 17). Lymphocytes with multidrug resistance and prominent numbers of B-cells are parameters for a more resistant, steroid nonresponsive rejection episode. From a treatment perspective, A3 and A4 ACR is uniformly treated, while A1 ACR is usually ignored or followed clinically. The significance of A2 rejection is debatable. In addition, treatment options are guided to an important extent by the clinical situation and measurable changes of pulmonary function parameters like FEV1 or FEF 25–75 (19).

Actual follow up of patients after lung transplantation

Although transbronchial biopsy is highly specific and sensitive in the diagnosis of acute rejection after lung transplantation and side-effects are tolerable, indications for this invasive procedure must reflect clinical concerns and the reasonable expectation of changing management as a result of such change. Our monitoring of rejection episodes is based on pulmonary function parameters like FVC, FEV1, FEF 25-75 which are determined easily and daily by the use of home spirometry and by the clinical state of the patient. If FEV1 declines more than 10% from the individual baseline or clinical signs of rejection/infection are present further examinations including bronchoscopy with transbronchial biopsy are performed Routine rejection and infection diagnosis is based on pulmonary function measurements (i.e., FVC, and FEV1) which should be performed daily. In case of deterioration of lung function tests from an individual baseline, clinical signs of graft deterioration like malaise, elevated temperature, decreased exercise capacity and dyspnea or radiographic abnormalities, bronchoscopic examinations with or without transbronchial biopsies are necessary for diagnosis of infections and/or rejection. Concerning the incidence of acute rejection episodes after lung transplantation and the possibility for reliable non-invasive rejection monitoring by the clinical state of the patient (well-being, temperature, dyspnea), pulmonary function measurements and radiographic examinations, the use of routine bronchoscopic surveillance cannot be justified beyond the first 3 postoperative months, either by risk/benefit or cost/benefit comparisons. The intensity of antirejection therapy is based more on clinical signs and the deterioration of pulmonary function than on the histological grade of rejection except for grades A3 and A4.

Infection after lung transplantation

Introduction

Infectious complications are the main cause of early morbidity and mortality in heart-lung and lung transplantation. According to the report of the Registry of the International Society for Heart and Lung Transplantation, infections were the single most important cause of death and responsible for about 40% of all deaths in lung allograft recipients (22, 23).The incidence of infections correlates with the intensity of the postoperative immunosuppressive regimen. However, for a number of reasons infections differ from those occurring in other solid organ transplantation.

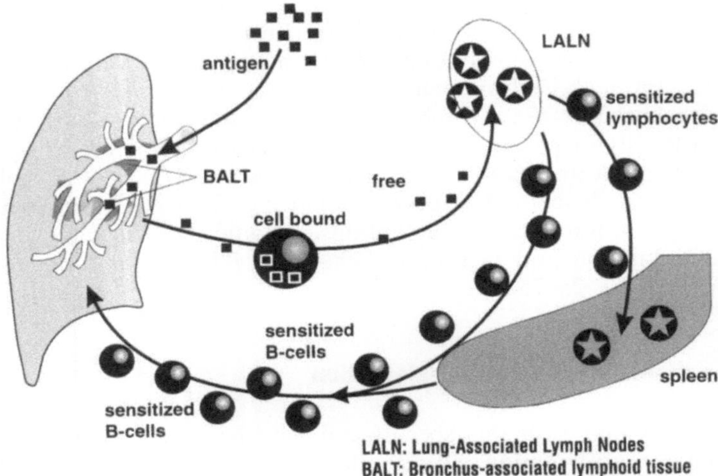

Fig. 8. Primary antibody response against intrapulmonary antigens - Uptake of antigens by the BALT across the epithelium - Immunoproliferative response in the LALN - Emergence of sensitized B-cells, which migrate and localize into the BALT

First, lung transplantation is, under the best of circumstances, a contaminated procedure. The transplanted lung is frequently colonized during donor management, recipients may suffer from chronic suppurative bronchial disease, the surgical opening of donor and recipient airways increases the risk of contamination of the surgical field, and donor and recipient commensal germs may cause post-operative pneumonitis.

Second, because of communication of the graft with the external environment, aerocontamination is more likely in lung transplantation.

Third, the transplanted organ by itself is the main target of infections and as a consequence, infection may frequently mimic rejection and may result in diagnostic and therapeutic errors. Moreover infection may promote rejection and/or obliterative bronchiolitis.

Fourth, recirculation of lymphocytes through the bronchoalveolar lymphoid tissue (BALT) is decreased in allografted lungs. Therefore the antigen uptake into the BALT from the airways is very low. Antigen uptake and transportation to the draining lymph nodes and the lung associated lymph nodes (LALN) is important for an adequate immune response, because antigen responses to infectious agents are primarily generated in the draining lymph nodes of the lungs. Additionally, the local immune response in BALT during viral infection is inadequate in transplanted lungs (Fig 8).

Perioperative prophylaxis of infection

To avoid early infections after lung transplantation high-dose, broad spectrum antibiotic and antimycotic therapy is necessary. Additionally, blood products should always be CMV negative and blood transfusions are performed with leucocyte filter systems to reduce the risk of leucocyte- transmitted viral disease. In our institute early antibiotic prophylaxis consists of the intravenous application of Clindamycin (600mg q.i.d.) which is active against a broad spectrum of gram positive bacteria as well as against anaerobes, Ceftazidime (2 g t.i.d.) with good activity against gram negative bacteria and especially against most of *Pseudomonas spp.* combined with Tobramycin

(3–5 mg/kgbw, single dose).To reduce the risk of aerocontamination by bacteria and fungal spores *(Aspergillus spp.)* all patients receive Tobramycin (80 mg) and Amphotericin B (10 mg) diluted in 2 ml NaCl 0.9% each per inhalation every 8 h (t.i.d.). Antibiotic therapy and antifungal therapy is continued at least for 10 days. Modifications of this protocol are performed if agents are cultured from the donor lungs or from the upper airways of the recipient which are not treated in an optimal way by this regimen. With this antibiotic and antimycotic regimen, combined with frequent bacterial and fungal examinations of wound and bronchial secretions, early infections after lung transplantation could be avoided nearly completely.

Opportunistic infections after lung transplantation

As in other solid organ transplantation opportunistic infections after lung transplantation are the consequence of immunosuppression.

In recent years, great progress has been made in the understanding of immune mechanisms for the host defense of bacterial, fungal , protozoal and viral agents.

Herpes viruses like *Cytomegalovirus* and *Epstein-Barr Virus* as well as the fungus *Cryptococcus neoformans* (24) and the protozoal agent *pneumocystis carinii* are mostly controlled and defended by T-cells, whereas the defense of *Legionella spp., Listerella monocytogenes* and *Aspergillus spp* is dependent on a sufficient number and adequate activity of macrophages and monocytes (25–31). *Toxoplasma gondii* and *Candida* defense is dependent on both the T-cell- and monocyte-macrophage systems.

The kind of immunosuppression applied and the exposure to environmental agents are the main determinants of the relative risk for primary or reactivated infection after lung transplantation.

To avoid infection and disease after lung transplantation preemptive therapies with antibiotic, antiviral and antiprotozoal drugs and adequate infection control measurements must be instituted.

CMV: CMV infection is the most frequent viral infection after transplantation, but symptomatic ones, and particularly pneumonitis, are more often observed in lung transplantation than in other solid organ transplantation. There are three major epidemic patterns of CMV infection in transplant recipients, each with its own rate of clinical illness.

First, primary CMV disease occurs when the transplant patient has no pretransplant experience with the virus (and is seronegative for CMV pretransplant) and is infected with virus carried latently in cells from a seropositive, latently infected donor, which is the source of infection more than 90% of the time. In the remainder, viable leukocyte-containing blood products from seropositive donors are the source of primary infection.

The *second* major epidemiologic pattern of CMV infection posttransplant is that of reactivation disease in which the transplant recipient who has been infected with CMV preciously (and is seropositive for CMV before transplantation) reactivates endogenous latent virus. The relative risk for reactivation of CMV-infection depends upon the type of immunosuppression used. It is obvious that cytolytic agents are the most important risk factors for virus replication and reactivation of disease, whereas cyclosporine A, FK506, rapamycine or prednisolone, administered without cytolytic drugs appear to have only minimal effects in term of reactivating latent CMV(32–36).

The *third* major epidemiologic pattern of CMV infection posttransplant is superinfection. The occurrence of this kind of infection depends on the natural exhibition of considerable genomic and antigenic heterogeneity of human CMV isolates (37).

Beside the direct viral cytopathogenic effect, the host's immune reaction triggered by the virus may cause pulmonary damage by enhancing the expression of MHC class I antigens on epithelial or endothelial cells (38). This may promote graft rejection, producing a protein homologous to MHC class I antigens and releasing potentially dangerous cytokines. Similarly to clinical observations in bone marrow transplanted patients, CMV pneumonitis may progress, regardless of the disappearance of the virus in the lung. Therefore, increasing the dose of steroids may sometimes be the option of choice for treatment of this kind of interstitial pneumonia.

To avoid infection and disease after lung transplantation, preemptive therapy including antibiotic, antiviral, and antiprotozoal drugs and regular monitoring of infection has to be instituted. Contrary to prophylactic therapy given to every patient at definite time intervals, preemptive therapy is a kind of treatment to prevent diseases guided by laboratory findings and clinical circumstances, which are strong indicators for a high rate of disease if the natural course of the infection is not stopped by an adequate therapy.

Our current regimen for the prevention and preemptive therapy of CMV infection after thoracic transplantation is based on an early application of gancyclovir in CMV-positive recipients or donors and on the early reinstitution of this antiviral therapy if virological parameters of CMV-replication like early antigens - for example pp65- and the CMV-DNA in peripheral lymphocytes are present or cytolytic therapy is necessary for rejection treatment in a CMV-positive recipient or with a CMV positive lung allograft (39) (Fig 9).

In lung transplant recipients it is important to note that contrary to the case with heart or liver transplant recipients, the cytomegalovirus can persist and replicate in the lung allograft without inducing viremia which can be detected by the early antigen CMV-matrix protein pp65 or the CMV-genome by PCR in peripheral blood mononuclear cells.

Since CMV infection and disease usually induce an immune response which is characterized by an increase of CD8 + T-cells and natural killer cells (NK), changes in the peripheral blood cells may be a possibility to get information about the dynamics of CMV infection which can indicate donor-transmitted primary CMV infection or CMV-reactivation in a CMV-positive recipient. It is important to initiate

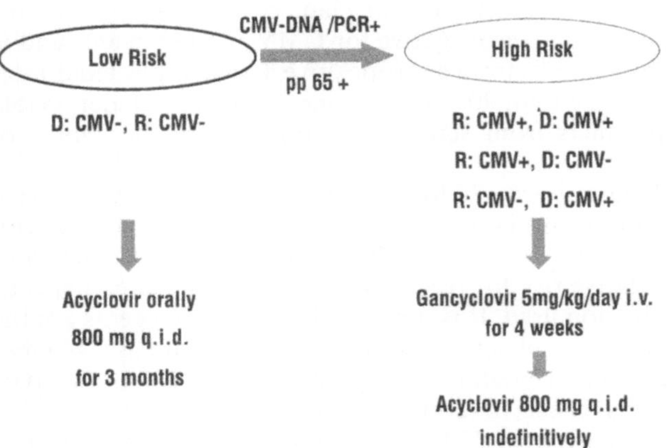

Fig. 9. Prevention and treatment of cytomegalovirus infection after lung transplantation

early preemptive therapy with gancyclovir (5mg/kg) once the change in the CD4/CD8 ratio is observed and before CMV-viremia or symptoms of illness becomes detectable.

Additionally, other immunological parameters can give an impression of the recipients's capability for an adequate immune response against bacterial, fungal, protozoal or viral agents. One distinct factor is HLA-Class II antigen (HLA-DR) which is expressed dynamically on the cell surfaces of lymphocytes and mononuclear cells. Measurements of the degree of HLA-DR expression can be done quickly on a day-to-day basis through flow cytofluometry (FACS) by use of monoclonal antibodies directed against epitopes of T-cells.

The usefulness of a combined view of bacteriological and virological examinations as well as of the immunological response in the transplant recipient to infections as determined by functional and numeric changes of mononuclear peripheral blood can be demonstrated by the course of a 56-year-old CMV-negative male heart-lung recipient, who received the heart and lungs from a CMV-positive donor (Fig 10). For the first 56 days CMV-prevention was achieved by administering 5 mg/kg bw gancyclovir. In the early phase HLA-DR expression on peripheral monocytes was high, reflecting a sufficient immune response to infectious agents. During pneumonia caused by *Pseudomonas spp.*, HLA-DR expression dropped to below 30%, indicating insufficient immune response, often referred to as immunoparalysis. Interestingly, at the same time the CD4/CD8-ratio changed from 15 to 0.1, indicating viral infection. The coincidence between the decrease in HLA-DR expression and the development of an inverse CD4/CD8 ratio may be accidental or, more likely, a consequence of the diminished cellular immune response to the bacterial infection.

Virustatic therapy was instituted again although there were no clinical signs or virological markers of CMV infection at that time. However, CMV infection was confirmed 1 week later by the proof of CMV-DNA in peripheral blood lymphocytes by PCR. A week later, antibodies against cytomegalovirus were detected. Because of the early initiation of preemptive antiviral therapy, which was indicated by the numeric and functional changes of peripheral blood cells the patient did not develop CMV-disease.

Some bacterial and fungal infections can also be prevented by preemptive therapeutic strategies.

Legionella infection: In our hospital, we have to use water from a water supply system which is colonized by *legionella spp.* Therefore *legionella* infection and especially *legionella* pneumonia has been a serious threat for transplant recipients.

Diagnosing *legionella* infections is difficult because *legionella spp* requires a special culture medium for growth and detection can be impossible if the culture media becomes overgrown with other bacteria. The antigen response to *legionella* infections is delayed in immunosuppressed patients (Fig. 11). We therefore initiated a legionella surveillance program in all transplant recipients whereby their urine was examined at least once a week for the presence of legionella antigens. *Legionella* antigens in urine are a highly sensitive marker for *legionella* infections and are detectable before the disease develops (40). In cases in which the *legionella* antigen was identified in urine, preemptive antibiotic therapy with erythromycin was capable of preventing *legionella* disease in almost all of our transplant recipients. Interestingly, we could detect *legionella* antigen in some patients for more than six months, an indication of the long time persistence of this intracellular pathogen under immunosuppression.

Aspergillus infection: Invasive aspergillosis is a matter of major concern after lung transplantation. Although this fungal infection occurs in only approximately 5–8% of cases in large transplant series, it is responsible for nearly 12% of deaths after single

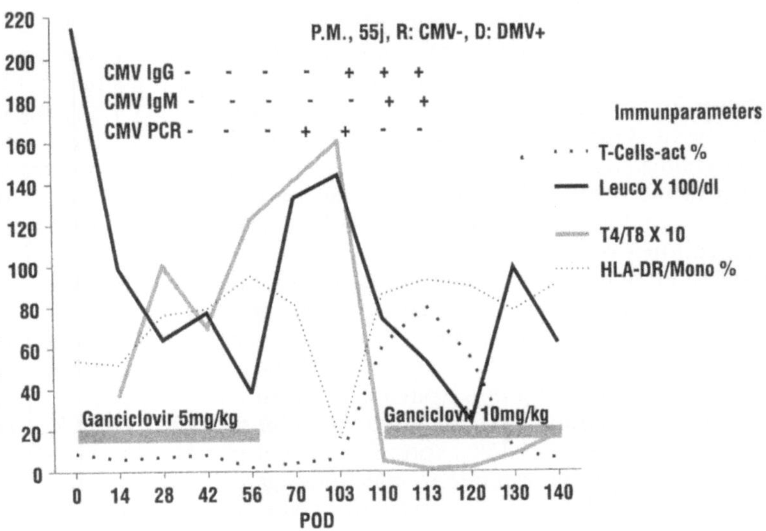

Fig. 10. Primary cytomegalovirus infection of a CMV-negative recipient who received a CMV-positive donor organ.
Course of leukocytes, activated T-cells, ratio of CD4 + /CD8 + T-cells, percentage of HLA-Class II (DR) positive monocytes after heart-lung transplantation

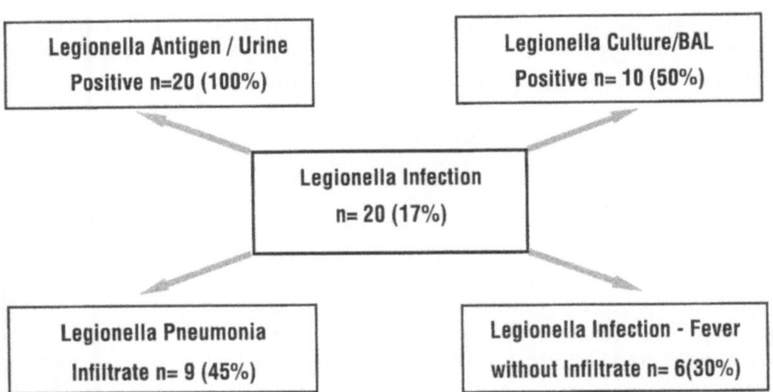

Fig. 11. Legionella infection after thoracic transplantation - incidence 17% ($n = 115$).
Sensitivity of Legionella antigen urine for Legionella infection 100%
Sensitivity of Legionella culture for Legionella infection 50%
Incidence of Legionella infection with fever but without infiltrate 30%
Incidence of Legionella infection with pulmonary infiltrate 45%

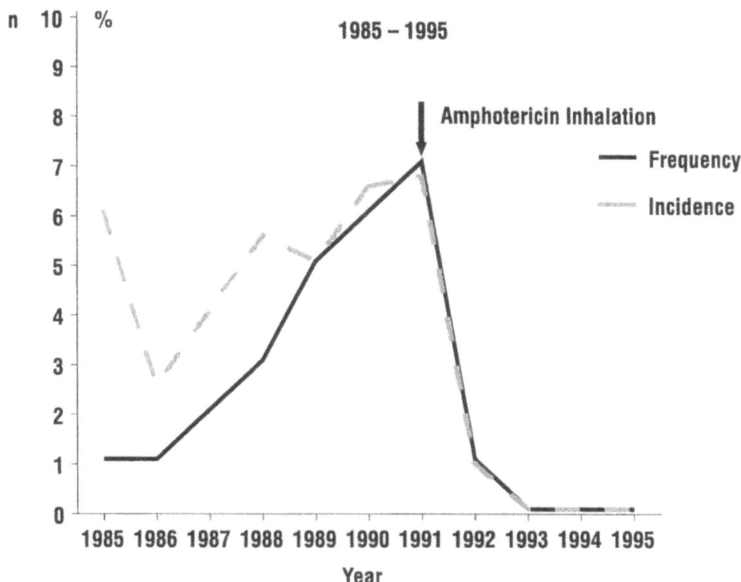

Fig. 12. Invasive aspergillosis after thoracic transplantation – Reduction of the incidence after preemptive therapy by inhalation of Amphotericin B

lung transplantation. In contrast to candidiasis, this fungal infection is airborne (41). After colonization of mucous membranes by *Aspergillus*, in connection with a certain predisposition of patients, invasive growth mainly occurs in the lung and sometimes in the paranasal sinus. A weakness in cellular immunity after administration of CyA, AZA, prednisolone, ATG, ALG, or OKT3-ab shortly after transplantation favors a very fast tissue invasion (42, 43, 44). Preemptive therapy is particularly necessary for this dangerous infection because its cure is rarely possible in transplanted lungs early after transplantation (45). In addition to exposure prophylaxis to fungal spores and frequent mycological examinations of sputum and bronchial secretions, we have introduced a preemptive therapy involving the inhalation of amphotericin B 10 mg t.i.d., which is begun immediately after transplantation and continued until the patient is discharged about 8 weeks after transplantation and later on, in case of rejection therapy. The rationale for this therapy is to enhance the phagocytic capacity of alveolar macrophages for *Aspergillus* spores and hyphae by incorporating amphotericin B into the lysosomes of alveolar phagocytes. Compared to intravenous administration, this type of preemptive therapy has the advantage that inhaled amphotericin B is not absorbed and therefore cannot cause systemic side effects, such as hepatotoxicity and nephrotoxicity. Since the introduction of this preemptive therapy in 1991, we have observed a decisive reduction in morbidity and mortality after thoracic transplantation (Fig 12).

Conclusion

In conclusion, rejection and infection remain frequent and serious complications after lung transplantation. However, better rejection diagnosis and probably better immunosuppressive strategies, including new immunosuppressive drugs, such as rapamycin and mycophenolic mofetil which will become clinically available in the near future, represent promising advances in this difficult field of transplantation. On the other hand, increased knowledge about local and systemic immunological host defense mechanisms against infectious agents, infection diagnosis with higher accuracy, as well as adequate preemptive antibiotic, antifungal and antiviral therapeutic strategies can reduce the risk of infectious complications, and therefore, the incidence of morbidity and mortality decisively.

References

1. Yousem SA, Dauber JA, Keenan R, Paradis IL, Zeevi A, Griffith BP (1991) Does histopathological acute rejection in lung allografts predict the development of bronchiolitis obliterans. Transplantation 52: 306–309
2. Yousem SA, Berry GJ, Brunt EM et al. (1990) A working formulation for the standardization of nomenclature in the diagnosis of heart and lung rejection: lung rejection study group. J Heart Lung Transplant 9: 595–601
3. Prop J, Wildevuur CRH, Nieuwenhuis P (1985) Lung allograft rejection in the rat. II. Specific immunological properties of lung grafts. Transplantation 40: 126–131
4. Prop J, Wildevuur CRH, Nieuwenhuis P (1985) Lung allograft rejection in the rat. I. Accelerated rejection caused by graft lymphocytes. Transplantation 40: 25–30
5. Prop J, Wildevuur CRH, Nieuwenhuis. (1985) Lung allograft in the rat. III. Corresponding morphological rejection phases in various rat strain combinations. Transplantation 40: 132–36
6. Prop J, Kuiper K, Peterson AH et al. (1985) Why are lung allografts more vigorously rejected than hearts?. J Heart Transplant 4: 433
7. Hummel M, Kuhn M, Bub A, Bittner H, Mann B, Schneider B, v. Eickstedt KW, Forssmann WG, Hetzer R. Urodilatin (1993) a new therapy to prevent kidney failure after heart transplantation. J Heart Transplantation 12: 209–218
8. Nakhleh RE, Boleman RM III, Henke CA, Hertz MI (1991) Lung transplant pathology. A comparative study of pulmonary acute rejection and cytomegalovirus infection. Am J Surg Pathol 15: 1197–1201
9. Scott JP, Higenbottam TW, Clelland CA, Smyth RL, Solis E, Wallwork J (1991) A prospective study of 204 bronchoscopies in 52 heart-lung and lung transplant recipients using TBB. J Heart Transpl 10: 626–636
10. Trulock EP, Ettinger NA, Bruit EM, Pasque MK, Kaiser LR, Cooper JD (1992) The role of transbronchial biopsy in the treatment of lung transplant recipients. An analysis of 200 consecutive procedures. Chest 102: 1049–1054
11. Yousem SA, Paradis I, Griffith B (1994) Can transbronchial biopsy aid in the diagnosis of bronchiolitis obliterans in lung transplant recipients. Transplantation 57; 151–154
12. Rabinowich H, Zeevi A, Yousem SA et al. (1990) Alloreactivity of lung biopsy and bronchoalveolar lavage-derived lymphocytes from pulmonary transplant patients:correlation with acute rejection and bronchiolitis obliterans. Clin Transplant 4: 376–384
13. Yousem SA, Paradis IL, Dauber JH, Griffith BP (1989) Efficacy of transbronchial biopsy in the diagnosis of bronchiolitis obliterans in heart-lung transplant recipients. Transplantation 47: 893–896
14. Scott JP, Higenbottam TW, Sharples L, Clelland CA, Mullins P, Smyth RL, Stewart S, Wallwork J. (1991) Risk factors of obliterative bronchiolitis in heart-lung transplant recipients. Transplantation 51: 813–817
15. De Blic J, Peuchmaur M, Carnot F et al. (1991) Rejection in lung transplantation-an immunohistological study of transbronchial biopsies. Transplantation 2; 54: 639–644
16. Yousem SA, Curley JM, Dauber J et al. (1990) HLA-Class II antigen expression in human heart-lung allografts,. Transplantation 49: 991–995
17. Glansville AR, Tazelaar HD, Theodore J, Imoto E, Rouse RV, Baldwin JC, Robin ED (1989) The distribution of MHC Class I and II antigens on bronchial epithelium. Am Rev Respir Dis 139: 330–334

18. Clelland CA, Higenbottam TW, Monk JA, Scott JP, Smyth RL, Wallwork J (1990) Bronchoalveolar lavage lymphocytes in relation to TBB in heart-lung transplant recipients. Transpl Proc 22: 1479
19. Starnes VA, Theodore J, Oyer PE et al. (1989) Evaluation of heart-lung transplant recipients with prospective serial transbronchial biopsies and pulmonary function studies. J Thorac Cardiovasc Surg 98: 683–695
20. Otulana BA, Higenbottam T, Ferrari L, Scott J, Igboaka G, Wallwork J (1990) The use of home spirometry in detecting acute lung rejection and infection following heart-lung transplantation. Chest 97: 353–357
21. Millet B, Higenbottam TW, Flower CDR, Stewart S, Wallwork J (1989) The radiographic appearances of infection and acute rejection of the lung after heart-lung transplantation. Am Rev Respir Dis 140: 62–67
22. Lawrence EC, Holland VA, Young JB, et al. (1989) Dynamic changes in soluble interleukin-2-receptor levels after lung or heart-lung transplantation. Am Rev Respir Dis 140: 789–796
23. Hosenpud JD, Novick RJ, Breen TJ, Keck B, Daily P (1995) The registry of the international society for heart and lung transplantation: Twelfth official report - 1995. J Heart Lung Transplant 14: 805–15
24. Dauber JH, Paradis IL, Dummer JS (1990) Infectious complications in pulmonary allograft recipients. Clinics in Chest Medicine 11: 291–308
25. De Repentigny L, Petibois S, Boushira M, Michaliszyn E, Senechal S, Gendron N, Montplaisir S (1993) Acquired immunity in experimental murine aspergillosis is mediated by macrophages. Infect Immun 61: 3791–3802
26. Lyman CA, Walsh TJ (1994) Phagocytosis of medically important yeasts by polymorphonuclear leukocytes. Infect Immun 62: 1489–1493
27. Vecchiarelli A, Dottorini M, Pietrella D, Monari C, Retini C, Todisco T, Bistoni F (1994) Role of human alveolar macrophages as antigen-presenting sells in *Cryptococcus neoformans* infection. Am J Respir Cell Mol Biol 11: 130–137
28. Levitz SM, Dupont MP, Smail EH (1994) Direct activity of human T lymphocytes and natural killer cells against *Cryptococcus neoformans*. Infect Immun 62: 194–202
29. Hill JO, Aguire KM (1994) CD4 + T cell-dependent acquired state of immunity that protects the brain against *Cryptococcus neoformans*. J Immunol 152: 2344–2350
30. Denkers E, Gazzinelli R, Martin D, Sher A (1993) Emergence of NK1.1 + cells as effectors of IFN-v dependent immunity to *Toxoplasma gondii* in MHC Class I deficient mice. J Exp Med 178: 1465–1472
31. Gazzinelli RT, Denkers EY, Sher A (1993) Host resistance to *Toxoplasma gondii*, a model for studying the selective induction of cell-mediated immunity by intracellular parasites. Infect Agents Dis 2: 139–149
32. Rubin H (1990) Impact of cytomegalovirus infection on organ transplant recipients. Rev Infect Dis 12 (suppl 7): S754–S766
33. Calhoon JH, Nichols L, Davis R, et al. (1992) Single lung transplantation. Factors in postoperative cytomegalovirus infection. J Thorac Cardiovasc Surg 103: 21–25
34. Hutter JA, Scott J, Wreghitt T, et al. (1989) The importance of cytomegalovirus in heart-lung transplant recipients. Chest 95: 627–631
35. Maurer JR, Tullis DE, Scavuzzo M, et al. (1991) Cytomegalovirus infection in isolated lung transplantation. J Heart Lung Transplant 10: 647–649
36. Chou S (1986) Acquisition of donor strains of cytomegalovirus by renal-transplant recipients N Engl J Med 314: 1418–1423
37. Gundry JE, Lui SF, Super M, et al. (1988) Symptomatic cytomegalovirus infection in seropositive patients: Reactivation with donor virus rather than reactivation of recipient virus . Lancet 2: 132–135
38. Van Dorp WT, Jonges E, Bruggemann CA, Daha MR, van Es LA, van der Woude FJ (1989) Direct induction of MHC class I, but not class II expression on endothelial cell by cytomegalovirus. Transplantation 47: 469–472
39. Van der Bij W, van Dijk RB, van Son WJ, et al. (1988) Antigen test for early diagnosis of active cytomegalovirus infection in heart transplant patients. J Heart Transplant 7: 106–110
40. Horbach I, Hummel M, Fehrenbach FJ. Diagnostik der Legionellose bei Herztransplantierten. 1. Deutscher Kongress für Infektions- und Tropenmedizin. 1991. Kongressband. Abst. 236
41. Chaparro C, Maurer JR, Chamberlain D, Hoyos ADH, Winton T, Westney G, Kesten S (1994) Causes of death in lung transplant recipients. J Heart Lung Transplant 13: 758–766
42. Schaffner A (1985) Therapeutic concentrations of glucocorticoids suppress the antimicrobial activity of human macrophages without impairing their responsiveness to gamma interferon. J Clin Invest 76, 1755–1764

43. Diamond RD (1983) Inhibition of monocyte-mediated damage to fungal hyphae by steroid hormones. J Infect Dis 147: 160
44. Schaffner A, Douglas H, Braude A (1982) Selective protection against conidia by mononuclear and against mycelia by polymorphonuclear phagocytes in resistance to aspergillosis. Observations on these two lines of defense in vivo and in vitro with human and mouse phagocytes. J. Clin. Invest. 69, 617–631
45. Hummel M, Thalmann U, Jautzke G, Staib F, Seibold M, Hetzer R (1992) Fungal infections following heart transplantation. Myocoses 35: 23–34.

Author's address:
PD Dr. med. Manfred Hummel
German Heart Institute Berlin
Augustenburgerplatz 1
13353 Berlin, Germany

Management of bronchial complications in lung transplantation

H.-J. Schäfers

Department of Thoracic and Cardiovascular Surgery, Homburg University Hospital, Homburg/Saar

Introduction

Airway complications have traditionally been a major source of morbidity and mortality following lung transplantation. The clinical success achieved by the Toronto group in the late 1980s was largely based on their concepts of prevention and treatment of these complications. Using a pedicled omental wrap around the bronchial anastomosis, a decreased prevalence of bronchial stenosis was reported (3, 14). Bronchial dehiscence as a consequence of full thickness necrosis was contained by omentum (14). If bronchial stenosis occurred, endobronchial silicone stents were used for airway maintenance (14).

Within the past years, concepts have undergone changes. The use of omentopexy has been omitted by most groups (1, 11, 15). In addition to silicone, also wire stents have been used for the treatment of bronchial stenosis (16, 19, 20). More recently, sleeve resection of stenotic airway segments following lung transplantation has been proposed (17). Bronchial complications are no longer a catastrophic event but rather have become a well recognized and in most instances treatable sequela of lung transplantation.

Prevalence of airway complications

In the early experience with single lung transplantation, bronchial complications occurred in 12 to 25% of the cases (5, 14). This prevalence is significantly higher than that reported for heart lung transplantation (7), most likely to the arterial collateral blood supply in the latter form of pulmonary transplanation. With the early form of en-bloc double lung transplantation, up to 50% of the patients developed lethal and non-lethal complications due to airway ischemia (13). It was mainly for this reason that bilateral sequental single lung transplantation was substituted for the en-bloc technique (9). Using the sequential approach, bronchial complications have occurred in a rate similar to that of unilateral transplantation. Currently, a prevalence of 4 to 10% is reported by some groups (4, 11, 15).

Between 1988 and 1995, 130 patients underwent 146 isolated lung transplants at the Hannover Medical School. Of these, 70 were unilateral (31 right lung transplants, 39 left lung transplants), in 76 instances bilateral lung transplantation was performed.

A total of 14 bronchial complications occurred in 222 grafts at risk (12 patients) for an overall prevalence of 6.5%. In three grafts, full thickness necrosis of the donor airway resulted in bronchial dehiscence. In nine grafts (eight patients) limited ischemia resulted in bronchial stenosis. There was no significant difference in the prevalence between unilateral versus bilateral transplantation (5/70 versus 9/152 grafts). More complications occurred with right pulmonary grafts than with left (9 vs. 5), even though this difference was not statistically significant. Interestingly the right intermediate bronchus appeared to be a predilection site and has remained so over time.

With increasing experience, the prevalence of bronchial complications has decreased significantly. Among the first 14 grafts, six developed a significant stenosis requiring intervention (i.e., stent). Based on experimental evidence and supported by this clinical observation, more attention was paid to maintaining bronchial microcirculation during the early postoperative period (15). Using early administration of corticosteroids, intraoperative and early postoperative heparin, and prostacyclin, the prevalence could be reduced significantly. In the second group of patients, only six complications occurred among 106 grafts at risk. In this group of patients, three bronchial dehiscences and two stenoses occurred in association with postoperative infections including *aspergillus* and methicilin resistant *staphylococcus aureus*. In addition, the administration of prostacyclin lead to occasional hemodynamic instability. In the subsequent group of patients (102 graft at risk), prostacyclin was omitted. Instead, amphothericin B and colistin or vancomycin were used as inhalative treatment. In this group, only two instances of bronchial stenosis occurred, both confined to the right intermediate bronchus.

Treatment of bronchial stenosis

Stents

Initially, endobronchial placement of custom-made silicone stents was used for airway maintenance following development of post-transplant bronchial stenosis (Fig. 1) similar to the approach used for palliation of benign and malignant airway stenosis (2, 14). The Dumon stent represents a valid alternative which is commercially available in many sizes (6). Expandable metallic stents are preferred by other groups (8, 19). Experience with this form of stenting has not been uniformly positive. Fractures have occurred with the early use of Gianturco stents (16), and reobstruction by protrusion of granulation tissue into the lumen of the stent has been reported (16, 19).

We have employed custom-made silicone stents in the treatment of six bronchial stenoses (five patients). The location of the stenotic segment was in the main bronchus in all instances (three right main bronchi, three left main bronchi). A total of 25 rigid bronchoscopies with implantation or revision of the silicone stent were necessary in these five patients. Recurrence of stenosis distal to the stent and dislodgement of the stent were the two main reasons for reintervention. Long-term airway maintenance was achieved in two grafts (6 and 7 years, respectively). One patient died from obliterative bronchiolitis with early onset 4 months postoperatively, three grafts (two patients) were retransplanted for progressive and complex airway stenosis in combination with obliterative bronchiolitis within 3 years of the primary procedure. All patients had to be maintained on regular inhalation of N-Acetyl-Cystein to prevent

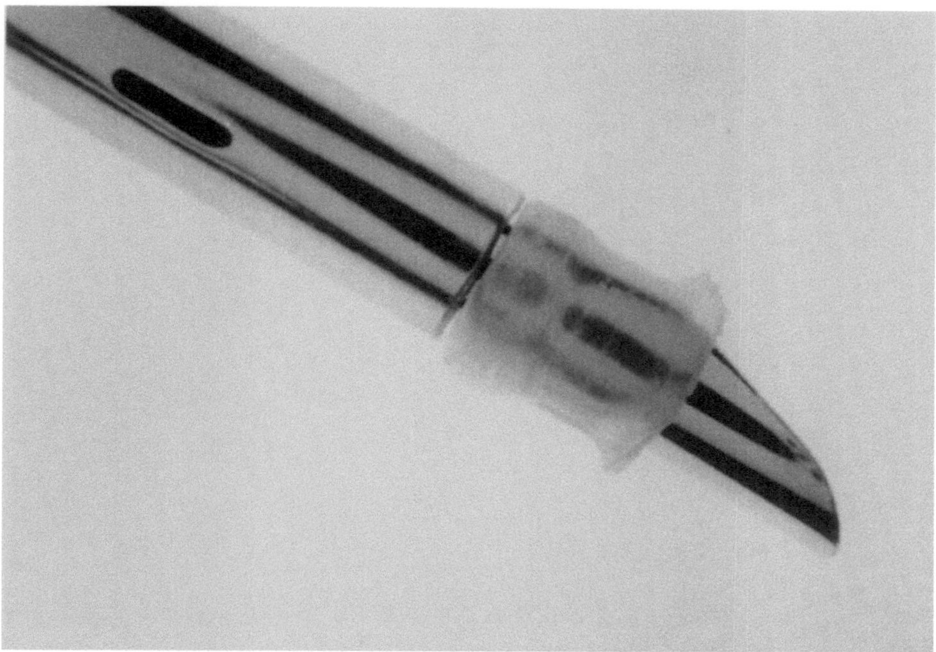

Fig. 1. Custom-made silicone stent mounted on rigid bronchoscope to be used for insertion into short left mainstem bronchial stenosis

retention of secretions within the stent. Six therapeutic bronchoscopies were required to remove partial obstruction of the stent due to secretions.

Our experience with self-expanding metal stents has been limited to three Gianturco stents, which were used in two heart-lung and one double lung transplant patients. One spontaneous fracture of the stent was observed (Fig. 2), and in the lung transplant patient progressive stenosis recurred due to tissue ingrowth. This latter patient ultimately underwent retransplantation.

Surgical Treatment

Since parenchyma-sparing bronchoplastic procedures have become routine in current thoracic surgery, a surgical approach to the treatment of posttransplant bronchial stenosis only appears logical. Up to our recent report (17), however, there were no publications describing operative reintervention for stenosis.

Our own experience started with a 48-year-old patient who developed stenosis of his right intermediate bronchus following double lung transplantation. Between follow-up bronchoscopies, the stenosis progressed to a point where a guide wire could not be passed into the distal airways and bronchoscopic management of this lesion appeared impossible. In view of his otherwise acceptable pulmonary function a decision was made to resect right middle and lower lobes. During the operation, multiple collateral vessels were found in the peribronchial tissue. The postoperative course was unremarkable and the patient continues to do well.

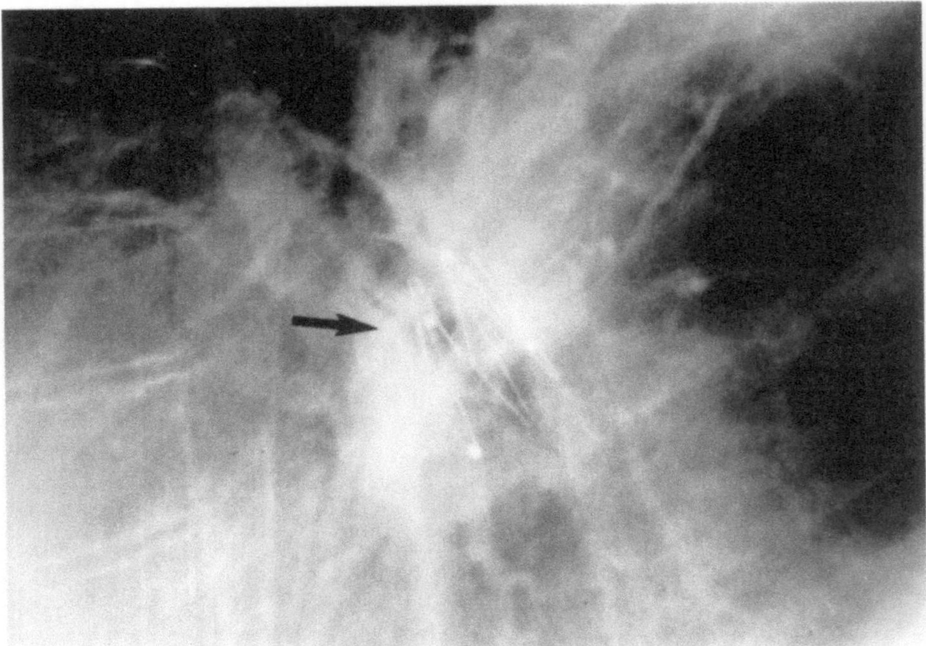

Fig. 2. Gianturco stent inserted for recurrent right main bronchial stenosis in a patient double lung transplantation. A fracture can be seen (arrow)

A second patient presented with stenosis of his left main and upper lobe bronchus following left lung transplantation (Fig. 3). Several attempts at placement of a Y-shaped stent failed. Thus, resection of the stenotic airway or retransplantation appeared as the only therapeutic alternatives. In view of donor availability, parenchyma-sparing sleeve resection of the stenotic airway was performed with reconstruction of the remaining lobar bronchi. The postoperative course was unremarkable and the patient continues to do well with patent airways two years following this procedure (Fig. 3B).

We have since then performed sleeve resection of stenotic graft airways in an additional three patients. In all three, stenosis of the right intermediate bronchus occurred following double lung (N = 2) or right lung transplantation (N = 1) (Fig. 4A, B). In all instances the extent of severe, postinflammatory adhesions was limited to the length of airway to be resected. The early postoperative course was unremarkable, all patients could be extubated within 24 h and discharged between 12 and 24 days postoperatively. All have had patent airways since, without further need for intervention.

Treatment of bronchial dehiscence

Extensive ischemia of the graft airway may result in full thickness necrosis and subsequent dehiscence of the airway. Operative revision and reanastomosis of the

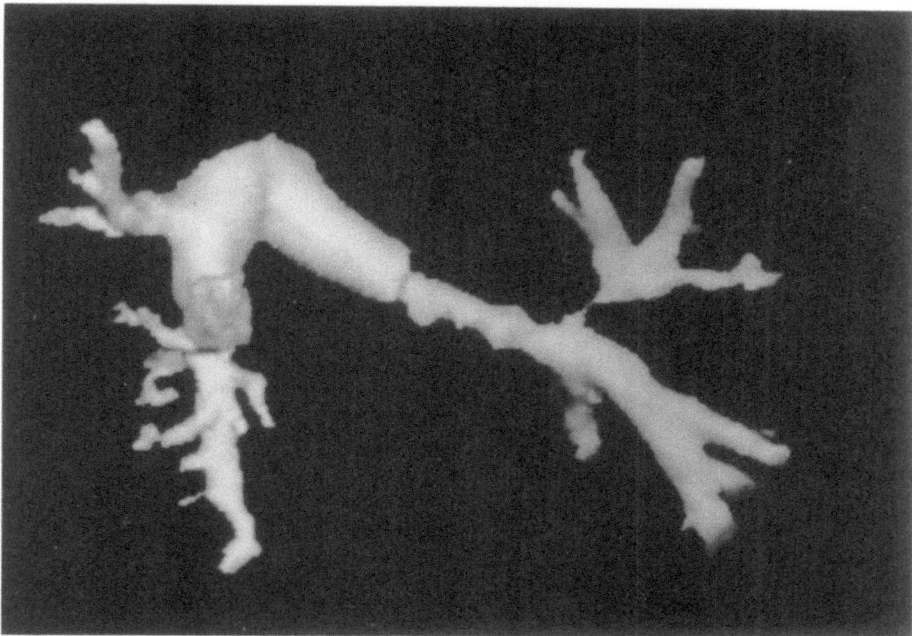

Fig. 3A. Three dimensional reconstruction of preoperative spiral computed tomography with visualization of central airways. There is a moderate long stenosis in the distal left main bronchus. The upper lobe bronchus is occluded. Normal airway dimensions are seen in lingula and apical bronchi. The lower bronchus appears normal

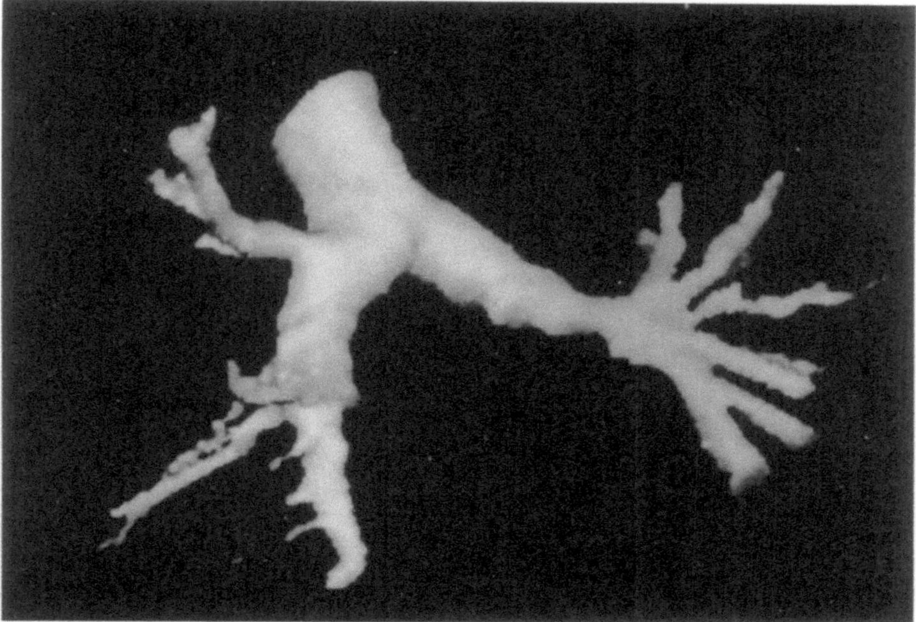

Fig. 3B. Reconstruction of postoperative spiral CT. There is mild narrowing at the site of the anastomosis. The superior segment of the lower lobe was been resected. The lobar and segmental bronchi are patent

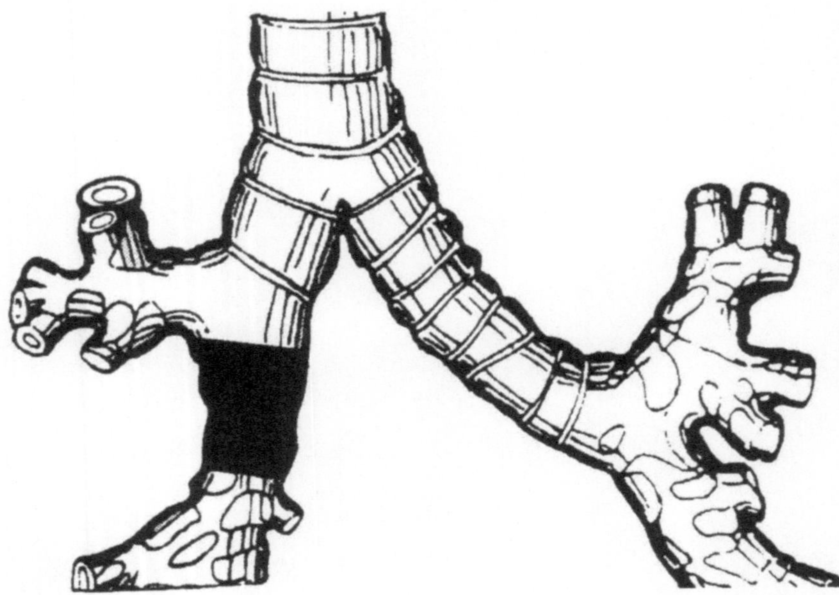

Fig. 4A. Operative approach for sleeve resection of the right intermediate bronchus. The stenotic segment extends from the central portion of the intermediate bronchus to the bronchial origins of middle lobe and superior segment of lower lobe

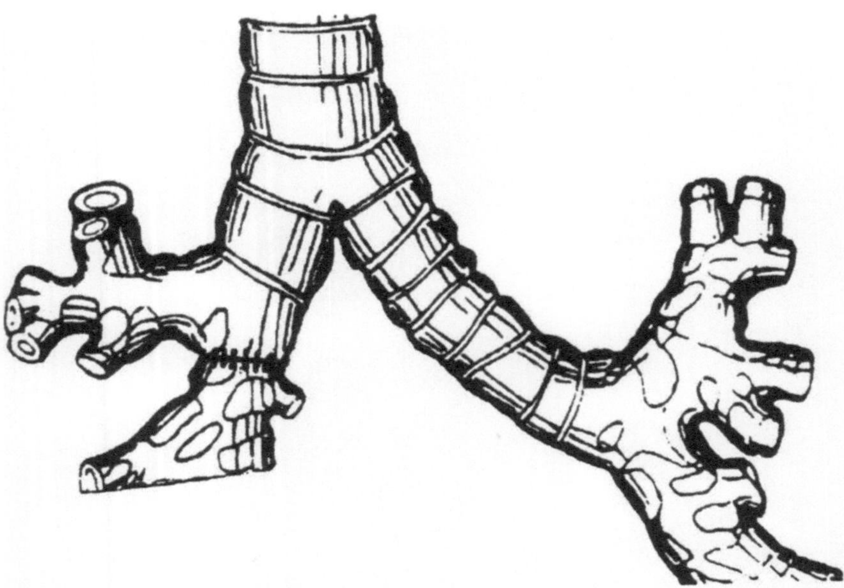

Fig. 4B. Schematic drawing of postoperative anatomy. The stenotic segment has been resected. The distal airways have been anastomosed to right main and upper lobe bronchi

bronchus has been used successfully in one instance (12). Retransplantation has been chosen by others with limited success (5, 13). Sudden massive hemoptysis from a bronchio-vascular fistula may occur and is almost uniformly lethal.

Our experience with dehiscence has been limited. In one instance, progressive necrosis of the graft right main bronchus occurred in conjunction with necrotizing bronchitis due to local infection with *aspergillus*. Reoperation and reanastomosis of the airways was performed; the patient, however, died from progressive sepsis spreading into the mediastinum. A second patient developed bilateral progressive bronchial necrosis in conjunction with local *aspergillus* infection. Eight weeks following his transplant procedure he developed a sudden episode of hemoptysis from erosion of his left pulmonary artery. He could be resuscitated and maintained on ventilation of his right lung with his left airways blocked. Emergency retransplantation was performed successfully. Ultimately, the patient died 2 years following retransplantation from progressive obliterative bronchiolitis.

Conclusion

With increasing experience and changing concepts, the prevalence of airway complications has decreased significantly after lung transplantation. Severe bronchial ischemia infrequently leads to complete disruption of the graft airways. While emergency retransplantation is an option, it is limited by the lack of available donors and possibly impaired medium-term prognosis after retransplantation with respect to graft function (21). Limited bronchial ischemia, as seen by surveillance bronchoscopy, occurs in approximately 20% of the grafts. In most instances this will heal without further intervention. Close observation with respect to the development of airway stenosis appears as reasonable primary option. Should bronchial stenosis occur, balloon dilatation via fiberoptic bronchoscopy can be employed for temporary relief (10); recurrence of stenosis following dilatation, however, is frequent or almost the rule. Other measures have to be taken to achieve long-term airway maintenance. Silicone stents have been used traditionally. Stent dislodgement, development of stenosis distal to the stented airway, and obstruction by secretions limit their use. Self-expanding metallic stents appear to have an advantage with respect to ease of insertion. The long-term results are limited by the possibility of tissue ingrowth through the mesh of the stent. Retransplantation is of only limited value in view of donor organ shortage and the possibility of accelerated development of obliterative bronchiolitis compared to primary transplantation. Resection of stenotic segments of donor airways is a new option which has so far resulted in excellent short- and long-term results.

References

1. Calhoon JH, Grover FL, Gibbons WJ (1991) Single lung transplantation. Alternative indications and technique. J Thorac Cardiovasc Surg 101: 816–825
2. Colt HG, Janssen JP, Dumon JF, Noirclerc MJ (1992) Endoscopic management of bronchial stenosis after double lung transplantation. Chest 102: 10–17
3. Cooper JD, Pearson FG, Patterson GA (1987) Technique of successful lung transplantation in humans. J Thorac Cardiovasc Surg 93: 173–181

4. Couraud L, Baudet E, Martigne C (1992) Bronchial revascularization in double-lung transplantation: a series of 8 patients. Ann Thorac Surg 53: 88–94
5. De Hoyos AL, Patterson GA, Maurer JR, Ramirez JC, Miller JD, Winton TL (1992) Pulmonary transplantation. Early and late results. J Thorac Cardiovasc Surg 103: 295–306
6. Dumon JF (1990) A dedicated tracheobronchial stent. Chest 97: 328–332
7. Griffith BP, Hardesty RL, Trento A (1987) Heart-lung transplantation: lessons learned and future hopes. Ann Thorac Surg 43: 6–16
8. Higgins R, McNeil K, Dennis C, Parry A, Large S, Nashef SAM, Wells FC, Flower C, Wallwork J (1994) Airway stenoses after lung transplantation: management with expanding metal stents. J Heart Lung Transplant 13: 774–778
9. Kaiser LR, Pasque MK, Trulock EP, Low DE, Dresler CM, Cooper JD (1991) Bilateral sequential lung transplantation: the procedure of choice for double-lung replacement. Ann Thorac Surg 52: 438–446
10. Keller C, Frost A (1992) Fiberoptic bronchoplasty. Chest 102: 995–998
11. Khaghani A, Tadjkarimi S, Al-Kattan K, Banner N, Daly R, Theodoropoulos S, Madden B, Yacoub M (1994) Wrapping the anastomosis with omentum or an internal mammary artery pedicle does not improve bronchial healing after single lung transplantation: results of a randomized clinical trial. J Heart Lung Transplant 13: 767–773
12. Kirk AJB, Conacher ID, Corris PA, Ashcroft T, Dark JH (1990) Successful surgical management of bronchial dehiscence after single-lung transplantation. Ann Thorac Surg 49: 147–149
13. Patterson GA, Godd TR, Cooper JD, Pearson FG, Winton TL, Maurer J (1990) Airway complications after double lung transplantation. J Thorac Cardiovasc Surg 99: 14–21
14. Schäfers HJ, Haydock DA, Cooper JD (1991) The prevalence and management of bronchial anastomotic complications in lung transplanation. J Thorac Cardiovasc Surg 101: 1044–1052
15. Schäfers HJ, Haverich A, Wagner TOF, Wahlers T, Alken A, Borst HG (1992) Decreased incidence of bronchial complications following lung transplantation. Eur J Cardiothorac Surg 6: 174–179
16. Schäfers HJ, Hamm M, Wagner TOF (1992) Gianturco self-expanding metallic stents. Eur J Cardiothorac Surg 6: 278
17. Schäfers HJ, Schäfer CM, Zink C, Haverich A, Borst HG (1994) Surgical treatment of airway complications after lung transplantation. J Thorac Cardiovasc Surg 107: 1476–1480
18. Schäfers HJ, Hausen B, Wahlers T, Fieguth HG, Jurmann M, Borst HG (1995) Retransplantation of the lung. Eur J Cardiothorac Surg 9: 291–296
19. Sonett JF, Keenan RJ, Ferson PF, Griffith BP, Landreneau RJ (1995) Endobronchial management of benign, malignant and lung transplantation airway stenoses. Ann Thorac Surg 59: 1417–1422
20. Spatenka J, Khagani A, Irviong JD, Theodoropoulos S, Slavik Z, Yacoub MH (1991) Gianturco self-expanding metallic stents in treatment of tracheobronchial stenosis after single lung and heart-lung transplantation. Eur J Cardiothorac Surg 5: 648–652
21. Schäfers HJ, Hausen B, Wahlers T, Fieguth HJ, Jurmann M, Borst HG (1995) Retransplantation of the lung. Eur J Cardiothorac Surg 9: 291–296

Author's address:
H.-J. Schäfers, M.D.
Department of Thoracic and Cardiovascular Surgery
Homburg University Hospital
66421 Homburg/Saar, Germany

Lung transplantation in cystic fibrosis

D. Metras[1], L. Viard[2], B. Kreitmann[1], A. Riberi[1], J.P. Chazalette[3],
J. Camboulives[2]

[1]Cardiothoracic Surgery, La Timone Children's Hospital, Marseilles (FR)
[2]Anesthesia and Intensive Care Unit, La Timone Children's Hospital,
Marseilles (FR)
[3]Renée Sabran Hospital, Cystic Fibrosis Center, Giens (FR)

Introduction

Until 1984, cystic fibrosis (CF) was considered as a contra-indication to lung transplantation for the following reasons: 1) The importance of the bronchopulmonary sepsis with polyresistant organisms inducing an increased post-operative risk. 2) The persistence of the native trachea and infected sinuses with a potential for mid-term additional septic risk in immunosuppressed patients. 3) The systemic aspect of the disease, with continuous pancreatic and hepatic evolving disease. 4) The unknown risk of constitution of the disease on the transplanted lung.

In spite of all these problems and the paradoxical aspect of the indications, heart-lung transplant in CF has been successfully performed in 1984 in Harefield (GB) (1) and thereafter in several US and European Centers (2, 3). Then, an important advance was brought by the concept of double-lung transplant (Toronto, 1987) (4), keeping the recipient's heart, and this was applied for the first time in a child in Marseilles in 1988 (5). Subsequently, several new and innovative approaches were described and used in CF patients: bilateral single lung transplant (6), lobar transplant from living donors (7), combined hepatic and lung transplant (8), etc.

A large number of these very sick patients were successfully transplanted worldwide, and the total number is now around 600 patients. The survival rate is variable with the series: 42 to 85% at 1 year, 23 to 76% at 2 years. A number of complications lead to the death of the patients: rejection, bronchiolitis obliterans, bacterial infections, viral infections in particular CMV, and often combination of two or more of these.

The present work will: 1) Discuss some aspects of the indications and controversies in CF patients. 2) Discuss the differential surgical approaches in this disease. 3) Analyze briefly the results based upon a French registry and our own experience in 35 pediatric transplants in CF patients.

Indications and controversies
of lung transplantation in CF

Cystic fibrosis (CF) is the most common lethal genetic disease in caucasians. The widespread disturbance of electrolytic transport and protein excretion in exocrine glands leads to pulmonary disease, exocrine pancreatic dysfunction with malabsorption and diabetes mellitus. Hepatic cirrhosis occurs also in 5 to 10% of the patients. In the last 10 years several advances have been made in the understanding of the disease: identification of the gene (9) and identification of the chloride channel abnormality (10). New therapies became available and continuous progress in the care of the patients has extended the survival to around 30 years. However, the most common cause of death is due to the effect of bronchiectasis with septic secretion, repeated infectious episodes with multiresistant pseudomonas, and finally terminal respiratory insufficiency. Therefore, before the time when genetic therapy can be instituted, probably within several decades, lung transplantation will be the only hope of survival for many CF patients.

Indication for transplantation needs obviously some criteria of acceptance, since only patients at terminal stage of the disease will be considered for transplantation. Most patients are followed and treated in specialized centers. They are therefore presented to the transplantation when a number of criteria have been reached despite intensive therapy:

General criteria of acceptance

They may vary with the centers, but a certain number of criteria are usually accepted (11):

Age less than 50 years
Life expectancy less than 12 months
No significant renal or hepatic failure
No evidence of malignancy
Ability to participate in rehabilitation program therapeutic compliance
Progressive decline of pulmonary function tests: FEV below 30% of predicted value.

Increasing frequency of respiratory infections leading to frequent hospital admis
sion for IV antibiotic treatment
Need for continuous oxygen therapy and/or use of nasal respirator at home

The Schawchman-Kulczycki scoring system (11) has been useful in children. The maximum is 100 points, below 50 it is considered as a strong indication for transplant.

All these parameters are not considered in isolation, but evaluated in the general patient and social context.

In the pre-transplant evaluation a precise cardiac assessment with echocardiogram and/or catheterization is done in view of the procedure chosen (bilateral lung transplant with conservation of the heart, heart-lung transplant (HLT) with or without Domino procedure.

The CF patient is obviously not an ideal candidate for transplant due to the continuous infectious process, the poor nutritional status despite maximum therapy including occasionally gastrostomy, jejunostomy, or parenteral supplementation, the presence of problems of irregular absorption of cyclosporin, etc.

However, due to their poor life with continuous medical environment, they are generally very aware of treatments, very compliant to therapy, and extremely in favor of transplant. We have seen this also in our pediatric population with strong parental support, and these factors are favorable for a transplantation decision.

Once the patient has been discussed between the cystic fibrosis specialists and the transplant team, and accepted for transplant, he usually is prepared actively and is ready to come urgently to the transplant center.

Special situations and controversies

There are many points of discussion and controversies in the difficult field of lung transplantation in CF. Some of these problems are briefly discussed below.

Previous history of thoracic surgery
In the first years of lung transplantation, this was considered as an absolute contraindication, in view of the operative hemorrhagic risk.

With the present approach, particularly with the clam-shell incision allowing excellent control of both chests, it is no more a contraindication for most teams (6, 11, 12). Pleurodesis and pleurectomy to treat repeat pneumothoraces may cause the worst difficulties.

Patients with multiresistant pseudomonas and cepacia regardless of its antibiotic sensitivity have been considered by some as contraindication to transplant
Currently however they seem to be accepted by most centers, due to the irreversible development of such bacterial harboring (11). The same accounts for the presence of *Candida* and *Aspergillus Fumigatus.*

Infected sinuses raise a problem of management
Preoperative drainage is useful in case of purulent retention, but the resection of polyps has usually been deceptive since they reccur rapidly, and we no longer perform repeated resection of nasal polyps, unless they are very important.

Other major organs and particularly hepatic dysfunction have been generally considered as a contraindication to transplant
However, several attempts at combined thoracic organs and liver transplant have been made (13) with a recent excellent series (8). However, this experience, we think, should be confined to experienced teams with an excellent multiorgan transplant environment.

Need for mechanical ventilation (MV) with intubation or tracheostomy was considered among the absolute contraindications to lung transplant in CF patients
As a matter of fact, once they are ventilated, most patients die within 2 or 3 weeks and, in spite of MV, elevated PC02 persist. Other organ failure invariably follows this situation.

However, provided no other organ fails, MV is no more considered *per se* as a contraindication to transplant (14). In our population of CF patients, mechanically ventilated patients were transplanted with a similar rate of success as the non-ventilated ones (15). Anecdotically, one of our pediatric retransplantations was tracheotomized and ventilated 66 days before successful retransplant (16). However, the situation is different if the patient is already on the waiting list when put on the ventilator or on the ventilator when seen for the first time by the transplant team. In general, it seems appropriate (17) not to consider the second situation as a transplantation candidacy since no evaluation and preparation has been possible.

Retransplantation
Retransplantation is a highly discussed topic. Some consider that it should not be done (18, 19) owing to the poor results and the scarcity of donors. As a matter of fact the lung retransplantation study (20) shows worse survival rates compared with first transplants.

Retransplantation should not be performed systematically for all failing transplants, but we think that in selected patients this possibility should not be refused. The etiology of lung failure, the age of the patients, the compliance and psychological assessment should be important factors to examine before taking this decision.

Technically, retransplantation is perfectly feasible, and in our experience pleural adhesions have been easy to liberate, and the intraoperative risk has been minimized. One of our retransplants is currently alive 4 years after the procedure.

Surgical approaches

Heart lung transplantation (HLT)

Initially the procedure of choice performed in cystic fibrosis (1, 21), it has been abandoned by many teams for CF who have switched to lung transplantation. However some very experienced teams continue to perform HLT in CF (3, 21), advocating better results, less airway anastomosis problems, need for continuous training for this kind of operation (3) and use of the recipient's heart for a Domino heart transplant (1). Due to the uniform recovery of temporary failing hearts after double lung transplantation in CF, we think these arguments are valid only if all hearts are used for Domino, which is certainly not the case. HLT has also been advocated in case of pediatric transplant, due to the easier tracheal anastomosis management in case of healing problem. Our recent experience and the experience of lung or even lobar transplant in small children (22) does not support this argument. CF still represents the indication for 15.4% of HLT according to the IHLTS (23), but it is not clear if this is the total percentage or the present percentage.

Double-lung transplantation (DLT)

The enbloc DLT was described by Cooper et al. in 1987 (24), with the main purpose of keeping a basically normal heart. However, this type of operation with the extensive mediastinal dissection, the period of cross-clamping of the recipient heart, and above all the complications of the airway anastomosis have practically led to other types of procedures. As a matter of fact, if the suture is done on the trachea, several lethal complications have been reported (25). A tentative attempt at improvement has been suggested and performed (26, 27) with separate suture of both bronchi with a better vascular supply, but still, several complications occurred (16).

En bloc DLT with tracheal anastomosis and bronchial artery revascularization has been successfully performed (28, 29), but in view of the following procedure, is probably very rarely done.

Bilateral single lung transplant (BSLT)

The BSLT (6, 11, 16) through the bilateral transversal antero-lateral thoracotomy ("clam-shell") approach is probably now the routine procedure in most centers. It has the main advantage of giving a remarkable access to both pleural cavities (Fig. 1) with easy liberation of the lungs, even in the presence of generalized pleural adhesions. We

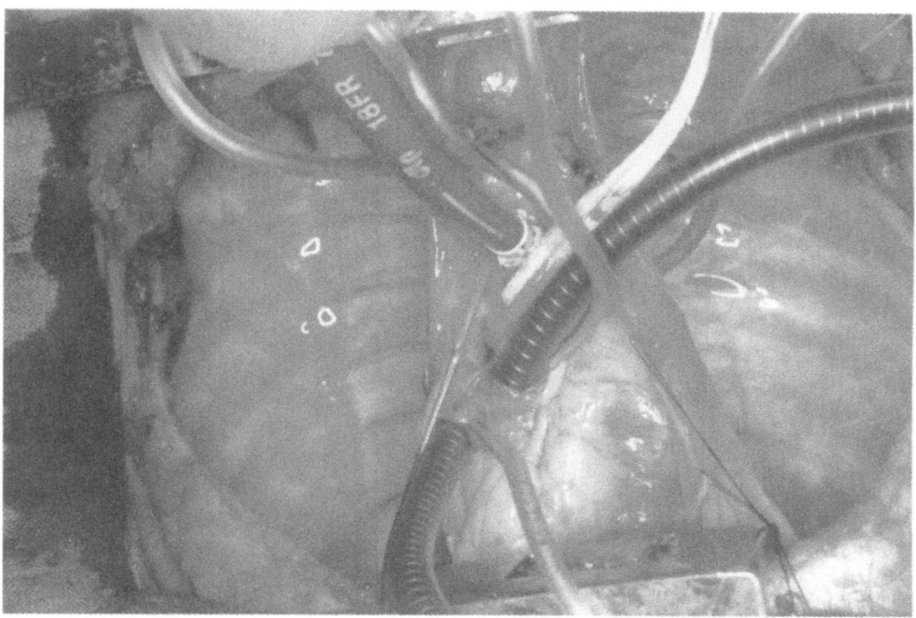

Fig. 1. Exposure by clam-shell incision, after lungs extraction in an 8-year old boy

have performed two redo BSLT with very little bleeding. Technically, two points deserve discussion.

Should CPB be avoided? Some teams have shown that it is possible to transplant both lungs consecutively without CPB and it has been advocated that bleeding and pulmonary dysfunction are avoided (11).

On the contrary, in pediatric transplant at least, but probably also in young adults, the use of CPB has not only been harmless, but also beneficial.

Due to the sometimes fragile hemodynamic condition, too much traction or retraction on large lungs may interfere with the cardiac function. Also, double lumen tracheal intubation is not available for small pediatric airways. Finally, with the frequent remote harvesting of lungs, to reduce the ischemic time, we routinely use CPB, remove the recipient lungs, prepare the stumps for anastomosis, and proceed to reimplantation as soon as the lungs are in the OR. To facilitate the dissection in a small chest and to avoid the presence of too many Satinsky clamps in the field, we place a gentle venting in the RV through the RA, clamp the main PA and the RPA with tourniquets and can divide both main PAs without clamps (Fig. 2). With this, there was little bleeding, and several patients had a bloodless procedure, four of them receiving no blood at all (Table 1) (17).

The lung function was satisfactory and in the last 14 BLST in children, the post transplant ventilation lasted from 1 to 7 days, with a mean cf 2.8 days.

Is bronchial suture safe and what kind of wrapping or revascularization should be done? It seems that a simple end-to-end anastomosis without any kind of wrapping or revascularization provide adequate healing even in children and babies as shown by several authors (22). It is interesting that still some continue to advocate telescoping suture (30) and omental wrapping (11). However it has been hypothesized that revascularization could improve long-term result and participate in the prevention of OB. This remains to be demonstrated.

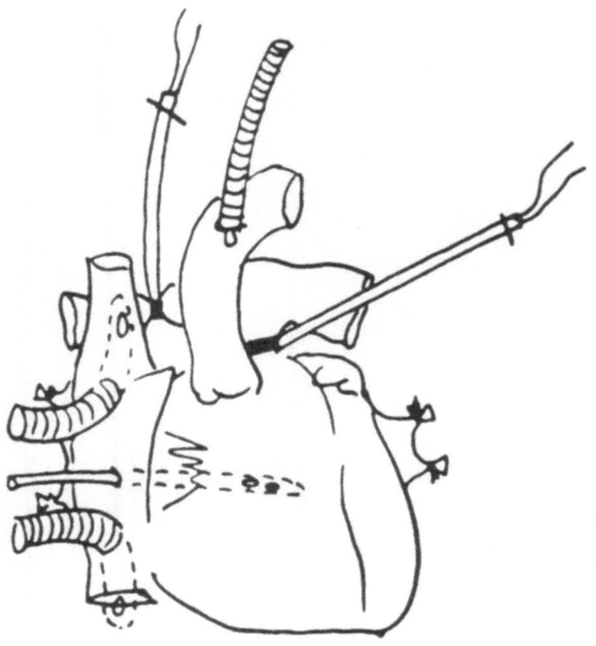

Fig. 2. Routine CPB used in BSLT with venting of the RV in a normothermic beating heart. Tourniquets on main PA and RPA allow division of both PAs without clamps

Table 1. Bleeding and transfusion

	Transfusion CPB (ml)	Transfusion after CPB (ml)	Transfusion 24 hours (ml)	Drainage 24 hours (ml)
En-bloc DLT (n = 10)	0 to 1000 (380)	0 to 800 (337)	0 to 200 (125)	730 to 5500 (1990)
Sequential BSLT (n = 24)	0 to 1350* (250) *oo*	0 to 1600 (260) +++	0 to 400 (240)	460 to 2900 (1050)

* Retransplantation   *oo* 10 pts without blood   +++ 4 pts without blood

Parenchymal reduction, lobar transplant, split lung

In view of the scarcity of donors in the pediatric group, a number of procedures has been advocated.

Harvesting of larger lungs is the simplest, and has demonstrated to be perfectly feasible: lobectomies (11), bilobectomies (16, 31) and atypical resection have been performed with results similar to other procedures. No particular complication has been noted. The parenchymal reduction can be accomplished *ex vivo* or after reimplantation.

Another possibility has been described: the splitting of the left lung into two lobes reimplanted on each side (31). This seems a very attractive procedure if only a larger left lung is available, and if the right lung is used in another transplantation. If not, the first procedure is probably simple.

The lobar transplant, particularly the living parental donor (7, 33) transplant, is a very fascinating option. However, apart from technical reasons, we think that the problem is mainly ethical: risk for the donor, psychological implications on the donors before the transplant, etc. At the present moment, with the "Bio-ethic law" in France (1994), this procedure is under evaluation.

Another conceptual problem is the future of a lobe if there is growth of the child. It is well known that after the age of 8 years, the number of alveoli is not going to increase and the future of an adult lobe is probably only a dilatation rather than growth.

Results

Early results

Early results have been continuously improving with time. In a large series of several centers in France, 180 transplantations have been performed in 168 patients (34).

The overall 6-month survival has increased from 51% before 1990 to 71.5% after January 1992. There has been no significant difference between HLT and BSLT in 3-month, 6-month, 1-year and 2-year survival.

However this difference was significant in patients below 10 years, and the survival was much worse (34). Presently in centers with experience in BSLT, the hospital mortality for a first transplant is extremely low, and sometimes zero (11, 16). The improved results in airway healing allows early use of steroids in the majority of the patients.

Mid-term and long-term results

Survival has been relatively rapidly decreasing in patients with initial successful transplantation for CF. Survival is between 55% and 65% (34) at 1 year in the French experience, and this is relatively similar to the international experience (23). Some centers however, have a better survival of 77% at 1 year (3) except for children under 15 years (35).

The patients recover a satisfactory lung function after 3 to 6 months to about 80% to 100% of the expected functional capacity (3, 6, 11) and their indices of satisfaction is elevated (3).

The cause of mortality is due to the usual problems of lung transplantation: rejection, infections, obliterative bronchiolitis and the combination of the three.

It is interesting to note that infectious episodes although frequent, are not more frequent than in LT for another etiology (3, 11).

A particular problem in our experience is the problem of CMV infection. In view of the scarcity of donors, of the frequent positivity of donors, and negativity of recipients, we have been obliged to cross the matching of CMV. Despite a continuous Ganciclovir prophylaxis and treatment of the infectious episodes, we have had a high mortality with CMV complications (16). It is interesting to note that some (11) have had frequent episodes of CMV infection with similar management and very few deaths (11). The efficacy of Ganciclovir has therefore to be questioned (11).

These complications have led in France in general (34) to a relatively deceptive rate of long-term survival (46% at 2 years since 1992 (34) and 28% at 5 years), and in our

Probability of graft survival*

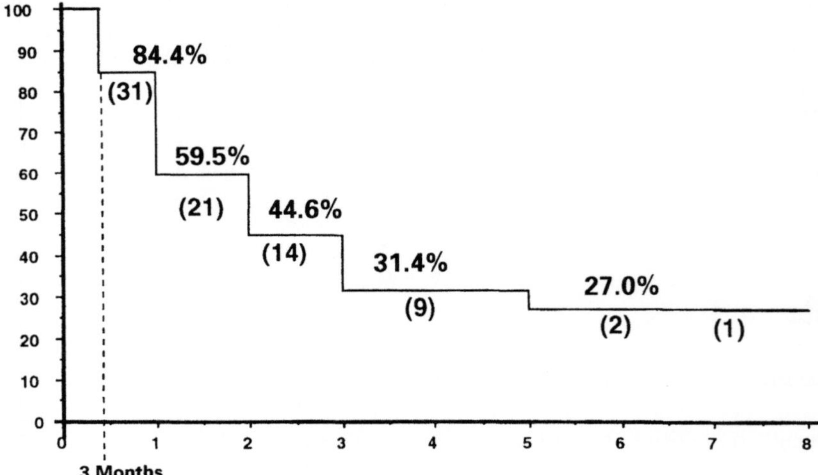

Fig. 3. Graft Actuarial Survival (N = 40). *The events are death of loss of graft

experience, in particular, (Fig. 3) 59.5% of graft survival, including death and loss of graft at 2 years, 44% at 3 years and 27% at 5 years).

Obliterative bronchiolitis remains a major cause of late death after LT in CF. The origin of OB is multifactorial but immunologic factors have demonstrated to be major contributors (35). It is interesting to mention that pediatric age is more prone to development of OB and non-compliance to treatment in this group is a possible factor (35).

The only option to counter the irreversible progression of OB is retransplantation with the drawbacks already mentioned (20).

Conclusions

The period of technical learning curve of all kinds of lung transplantations is about to be finished since the operative mortality has gone to a very low level.

However, LT in CF still represents a formidable challenge. The selection of patients, the numerous post-operative problems, infection being probably the greatest at mid-term, and bronchiolitis obliterans at long term, the scarcity of suitable donors represent major difficulties.

It seems that with the exception of LT at young age under 10 years, the results and complications of LT in CF have reached the same level as LT for other indications.

Therefore, although the results are somewhat disappointing, LT for CF should be continued as it is presently the only hope of survival in this dramatic disease.

Progress should be, we think, directed towards prevention and treatment of infection, particularly CMV, improvement in immunosuppression, and understanding of bronchiolitis obliterans.

Addendum

Although this chapter is delaing with a topic presented at a meeting held more than two years ago, the basic information still remains correct, it must be stated, however, that some centers have achieved more satisfactory results lately than the ones presented here with 5 years survival over 60% in adult population of patients.

Concerning children, despite the numerous problems encountered, transplantation still remains the best option for better and longer suvvival. Fig. 4 presents our experience (through 1997) with 60 children with CF presented for transplantation. The survival of the 34 that could be transplanted is significantly better than the survival CF of the 26 did not reach transplantation considering that all patients were accepted for transplant.

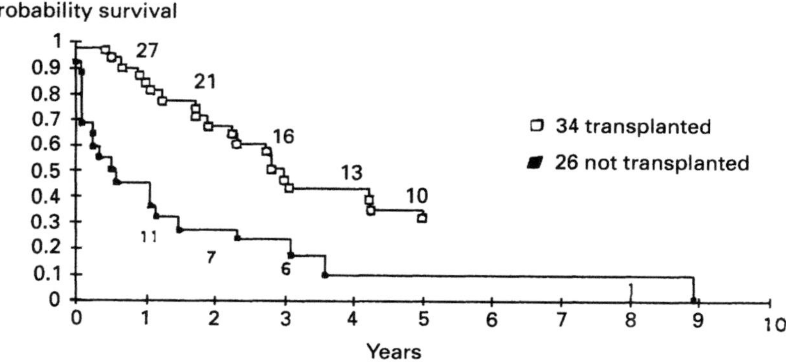

Fig. 4. Children with cystic fibrosis proposed for lung transplantation. Actual survival curve (Marseille Timone Hospital, 1988–1997)

References

1. Yacoub MH, Banner NR, Khaghani A et al. (1990) Heart-lung transplantation for cystic fibrosis and subsequent Domino heart transplantation. J Heart Transplant 9: 459–467
2. Frist WH, Fox MD, Campbell PW, Fiel SB, Loyd JE, Merrill WH (1991) Cystic fibrosis treated with heart-lung transplantation: North American results. Transplant Proc 23: 1205–1206
3. Dennis C, Caine N, Sharples L et al. (1993) Heart-lung transplantation for end stage respiratory disease in cystic fibrosis patients at Papworth Hospital. J Heart Lung Transplant 12: 893–902
4. Pasque MK, Cooper JD, Kaiser LR, Haydock DA, Triantafillou A, Trulock EP (1990) Improved technique for bilateral lung transplantation: rationale and initial clinical experience. Ann Thorac Surg 49: 785–791
5. Noirclerc M, Chazalette JP, Metras D et al. (1989) Les transplantations bipulmonaires: rapport de la première observation française et commentaires des cinq suivantes. AnnChir 43: 497–600
6. Ramirez JC, Patterson GA, Winton TL et al. (1992) Bilateral lung transplantation for cystic fibrosis. J Thorac Cardiovasc Surg 103: 287–294
7. Starnes VA, Barr ML, Cohen FA, Schenkel FA, Barbers RG, and the USC Transplant Group (1994) Nilateral living-related lobar transplantation for cystic fibrosis: initial experience (Abstract). J Heart Lung Transplant 13(Suppl): S57
8. Couetil JP, Houssin D, Dousset B, Loulmet D, Achkar A, Tolan MJ, Amrein C, Guinvarch A, Guillemain R, Birnbaum P, Carpentier A. Combined lung and liver transplantation in patients

with cystic fibrosis. A4 1/2-year experience. Read at the Seventy-fifth Annual Meeting of The American Association for Thoracic Surgery, Boston, Mass., April 23–26, 1995

9. Riordan JR, Rommens JM, Kerem B-S et al. (1989) Identification of the cystic fibrosis gene: cloning and characterization of complementary DNA. Science 245: 1066–1073

10. Knowles M, Gatzy J, Boucher R (1981) Increased bioelectric potential difference across respiratory epithelia in cystic fibrosis. N Engl J Med 305: 1489–1495

11. Egan M, Detterbeck FC, Mill MR, Paradowski LJ, Lackner RP, Ogden WD, Yankaskas JR, Westerman JH, Thompson JT, Weiner MA, Cairns EL, Wilcox BR (1995) Improved results of lung transplantation for patients with cystic fibrosis. J Thorac Cardiovasc Surg 109: 224–235

12. Metras D, Shennib H, Kreitmann B, Camboulives J, Viard L, Carcassonne M, Giudicelli R, Noirclerc M, and the Joint Marseille-Montreal Lung Transplant Program (1993). Double-Lung Transplantation in children: A report of 20 cases. Ann Thorac Surg 55: 352–357

13. Wallwork J, Williams R, Calne RY (1987 Transplantation of liver, heart and lungs for primary biliary cirrhosis and primary pulmonary hypertension. Lancet 2: 182–184

14. Flume PA, Egan TM, Westerman JH et al. (1994) Lung transplantation for mechanically ventilated patients. J Heart Lung Transplant 13: 15–21

15. Massard G, Shennib HH, Metras D, Giudicelli R, Camboulives J, Mulder J, Morin JF, Viard L, Noirclerc M (1993) Lung transplantation in ventilated patients with cystic fibrosis. Ann Thorac Surg 55: 1087–1092

16. Metras D, Kreitmann B, Riberi A, Viard L, Pannetier A, Garbi O, Marti JY, Noirclerc M (1995) Bilateral single-lung transplantation in children. Ann Thorac Surg 60: S578–S581

17. Shennib H (1995) P 84–87 in Lung Transplantation. Edited by GA Patterson, and L. Courand 1995; Elsevier Science

18. Madden BP, Hodson ME, Tsang V, Radley-Smith R (1992) Intermediate term results of heart-lung transplantation for cystic fibrosis. Lancet 339: 1583–1587

19. Smith J, Wallwork J (1995) Retransplantation in heart-lung recipient with obliterative bronchiolitis (letter). J Thorac Cardiovasc Surg 109: 818

20. Novick RJ, Andréassian B, Schäfers HJ et al. (1994) Pulmonary retransplantation for obliterative bronchiolitis: intermediate-term results of a North American series. J Thorac Cardiovasc Surg 107: 755–763

21. De Leval MR, Smyth R, Whitehead B et al. (1991) Heart and lung transplantation for terminal cystic fibrosis: A4 1/2-year experience. J Thorac Cardiovasc Surg 101: 633–642

22. Starnes VA, Marshall SE, Lewiston NJ, Theodore J et al. (1991) Hear-lung transplantation in infants, children, and adolescents. J Ped Surg 26: 434–438

23. The Registry of the International Society for Heart and Lung Transplantation: Twelfth official report-1993. J Heart Lung Transplant 14: 805–815

24. Patterson GA, Cooper JD, Goldman B et al. (1988) Technique of successful clinical double-lung transplantation. Ann Thorac Surg 45: 626–633

25. Patterson GA, Todd TR, Cooper JD, Pearson FG, Winton TL, Maurer J and the Toronto Lung Transplant Group (1990). Airway complications after double-lung transplantation. J Thorac Cardiovasc Surg 99: 14–21

26. Noiclerc M, Metras D, Vaillant A et al. (1990) Bilateral bronchial suture in double-lung and heart-lung transplantations. Eur J Thorac Cardiovasc Surg 4: 314–317

27. Metras D, Noirclerc M, Vaillant A, Brunet CH, Kreitmann B (1990) Double-lung transplantation. The role of bilateral bronchial suture. Transplant Proc 22: 1477–1478

28. Daly RC, Tadjkarim IS, Khaghani A, Banner NR, Yacoub MH (1993) Successful double-lung transplantation with direct bronchial artery revascularization. An Thorac Surg 56: 885–892

29. Couraud L, Baudet E, Nashef SAM, Martigne C, Roques X, Velly JF, Laborde N, Dubrez J, Clerc F (1992) Lung transplantation with bronchial revascularization. Surgical anatomy, operative technique and early results. Eur J Cardiothorac Surg 6: 490–495

30. Calhoon JH, Grover FL, Gibbons WJ et al. (1991) Single lung transplantation: alternative indications and technique. J Thorac Cardiovasc Surg 101: 816–825

31. Metras D, Shennib H, Camboulives J, Viard L, Carcassonne M, Giudicelli R, Silicani MA, Pannetier A, Garbi O, Geigle P, Marty JY, Badier M, Dumont JF, Chazalette JP, Kreitmann B, Mulder DS, Tchervenkov C, Noirclerc M (1992) Lung transplantation in children. J Heart Lung Transplant 11(4): S82–S85

32. Couetil JP, Grousset A, Benaim D et al. (1994–95) Mise au point expérimentale de la bipartition pulmonaire avec transplantation lobaire bilatérale chez le chien et application en clinique humaine. Chirurgie 120: 512–517

33. Starnes VA, Barr ML, Cohen RG (1994) Lobar transplantation: Indications, techniques, and outcome. J Thorac Cardiovasc Surg 108: 403–411
34. Foucaud P, Bloch J, Lenoir G, Navarro J, et le groupe "Transplantation et Mucoviscidose". Transplantation pulmonaire et mucoviscidose. Les données du registre national. Vièmes Journées de Monaco, 20 Mai 1995
35. Whitehead B, Rees P, Sorensen K, Bull C, Higenbottam TW, Wallwork J, Fabre J, Eliott M, De Leval M (1994) Incidence of obliterative bronchiolitis after heart-lung transplantation in childen. J Heart Lung Transplant 13: 903–980

Authors' address:
Prof. Dominique Metras
Université de Marseille
Hopital d'Enfants de la Timone
Service de Chirurgie Thoracique et Cardio-Vasculaire
13385 Marseille, France

Lung transplantation for acute pulmonary failure

A. Haverich, S. W. Hirt, M. Strüber, J. Cremer, W. Harringer, P. Dütschke[1],
J. Wawersik[1]

Dept. of Cardiovascular Surgery, Kiel University Hospital
[1]Dept. of Anaesthesiology, Kiel University Hospital

Introduction

Lung transplantation as well the combined replacement of the heart and both lungs could be established as a routine procedure at many cardiac surgical units during the last decade. Meanwhile, transplantation of the lung represents a realistic therapeutic option in a number of end-stage parenchymal and vascular pulmonary disorders. A prerequisite for lung transplant surgery is, however, the absence of transplant specific contraindications. With respect to the scarcity of suitable organ donors the potential recipient must, in addition, be able to survive a certain waiting time. Comparing with patients suffering from renal failure, who are able to survive endstage organ damage for many years using dialysis techniques, biotechnological bridging was impossible in severe heart or lung failure for many years. Recently, assist devices allow bridging in acute isolated lung failure for a certain period of time for either spontaneous recovery or subsequent lung transplantation. However, with respect to the enormous effort required in intensive care, medical costs and with respect to the donor shortage this therapeutic concept must be restricted to carefully selected cases.

"Elective" lung transplantation:
Indications and results

Indication for lung transplantation is given for endstage parenchymal and vascular pulmonary diseases in patients under 55 years of age, isolated single organ failure, dependent on oxygen, disabled in home activity, free of malignancy and without any further improvement under conventional medication. According to the registry of the International Society for Heart and Lung Transplantation, a total of 2428 heart-lung (HLTX), 4777 single lung (SLTX) and 3278 double lung procedures (DLTX) aside from 45 993 heart transplantations have been performed worldwide through March 1, 1998 (5). The actuarial 1-year survival is approximately 60% after HLTX, and 70% after both SLTX and DLTX (5). The increasing shortage of suitable donor organs results in an extended waiting time for transplantation of approximately 2–3 years within the Eurotransplant region. This represents the most limiting factor for patients suffering from end-stage lung disease and right heart failure. As a result, alternatives in medical treatment, surgery and emergency procedures are requested. With respect to the surgical procedure shaving of the lung has been re-introduced for selected cases of pulmonary emphysema (1). Also, with an increasing number of indications for isolated lung transplantation heart-lung transplantation is restricted to patients suffering from pulmonary hypertension secondary to an incorrectable congenital malformation (4). This allows to take care of 2–3 transplant recipients with a single thoracic organ donor.

Technique of extracorporeal oxygenation

In end-stage pulmonary failure, artificial ventilation requires a residual lung function and may result in additional damage to the lung. Often, recovery of the lung cannot be achieved by applying this conventional technique over a longer time period. Currently used techniques of artificial oxygen supply to the blood have resulted from the technical development of extracorporeal circulation (ECC) in open-heart surgery. Commercially available membrane oxygenators have recently allowed for safe oxygenation and CO_2 removal over a long time period without significant damage of the blood cells. Elimination of CO_2 ($ECCO_2$) does not represent a major problem in ARDS treatment using sufficient ECMO flow rates. The set-up of ECMO for bridging in acute lung failure is very similar to the heart-lung machine with an outlet and inlet line, a venous reservoir and especially in this utilization two membrane oxygenators, connected in parallel to allow for a quick change without interrupting blood flow. For cannulation in veno-venous ECMO, we place a long drainage cannula via the right femoral vein in the right atrium and for return of blood the right internal jugular vein is cannulated. Using the veno-venous technique pre-pulmonary oxygenation is generally sufficient in cases with isolated lung failure. In addition, the outlet resistance in the vein is lower than in the setting with arterial return resulting in reduced blood damage. Also, pre-oxygenation of the pulmonary artery blood is speculated to allow for better recovery of the damaged lung. The use of systems with complete heparine coated surfaces may reduce the risk of full heparinization especially in trauma patients, however, this setting does not allow the use of a venous reservoir (7). Alternative techniques such as intravascular oxygenation (IVOR) could not be established in clinical routine for bridging in severe lung failure due to the limited oxygen supply of this system when inserted into the inferior caval vein (6).

The combined approach: Indication and results

Two different patient groups are potential candidates for lung transplantation in acute pulmonary failure. The majority are patients listed for transplantation who are unable to survive the waiting time due to rapid deterioration. The second group are cases with acute pulmonary failure due to ARDS following trauma, operation, pulmonary infection or failed operative procedures in patients with pulmonary hypertension (e.g., failed pulmonary thrombendarterectomy). While in the first group spontaneous recovery seems to be unlikely the possibilty of recovery must be respected in ARDS patients.

Due to the shortage of organ donors lung transplantation in acute respiratory failure will be restricted to a small group of younger patients suffering from isolated pulmonary failure without contraindications for transplantation and free from ECMO related complications such as bleeding or infection. In agreement with their relatives the presumed consent of the patient has to be evaluated. On the other hand, indication for ECMO and subsequent lung transplantation may be given in selected cases of transplant candidates deteriorating during waiting time despite hospitalization and oxygen supply. In this subgroup, young patients suffering from non-infectious diseases and requiring unilateral lung transplantation should probably be preferred. This is in accordance with the fact that a single lung is much easier and sooner available in most circumstances. A duration of ECMO for more than 4 weeks is associated with an increased number of limiting complications. With respect to the presumed long waiting time for suitable heart-lung donor, therefore, candidates requiring heart-lung replacement are currently not acceptable for bridging with ECMO in our opinion.

The technique of extracorporeal membrane oxygenation has been established at many cardiac surgical centers for quite a long time. Nevertheless, the application of bridging in acute pulmonary failure is rare. With the introduction of lung transplantation as a routine procedure a realistic option was given for cases not recovering on ECMO. However, the necessity to obtain a suitable organ in time remains one of the major prognostic factors. In addition, the severe illness of the patients combined with threatening complications by ECMO and heparinization allow for only a limited time span for diagnostic evaluation. As a minimum, we always claim chest x-ray, broncho-scopy, cultures of bronchial aspirate, urine and blood for exclusion of extrapulmonary infection. Also, a cranial CT-scan for exclusion of intracerebral bleeding should be performed. One major problem in this group remains the unavailable patient consent, potentially resulting in ethical discussions.

Following a period of staged therapeutic interventions, patients suffering from respiratory insufficiency are first ventilated by use of specific techniques, and kinetic therapy is usually applied. In addition, application of nitric oxide, surfactant or C-1 esterase inhibitor may be necessary (Fig. 1). If this sequence of interventions is not successful, the indication for ECMO respectively lung transplantation is proved. Only then and in cases with unsuccessful weaning and missing contraindications for transplantation indication for lung replacement is discussed in suitable patients on an individual basis.

Table 1 gives our own experience in eight patients undergoing lung transplantation after various periods of extracorporeal membrane oxygenation for acute pulmonary failure. The duration of ECMO ranged between 1–40 (median: 5.5) days. The mean age of the five female and three male candidates was 32.5 $\pm$ 14.6 (11–54) years and underlying diseases were ARDS (n = 4), reperfusion damage after previous lung transplantation (n = 3), unsuccessful pulmonary thrombendarterectomy (n = 1). ARDS was caused in two patients by a traffic accident with severe thoracic trauma, in one patient due to unknown reason after kidney and liver transplantation. In an 11-year-old girl ARDS was precipitated by staphylocci pneumonia. In the last case no signs of systemic infections were present after approximately 3 weeks of ECMO and the girl was accepted for lung transplantation. In all cases standard treatment including mechanical ventilation, kinetic therapy, and application of various pharma-cologic agents such as nitrates, prostacyclin, NO, surfactant and C1-esterase inhibitor remained unsuccessful. Before application of ECMO, arterial oxygen tension ranged between 37 and 58 mmHg on 100% of oxygen. In a 23-year-old female, pulmonary

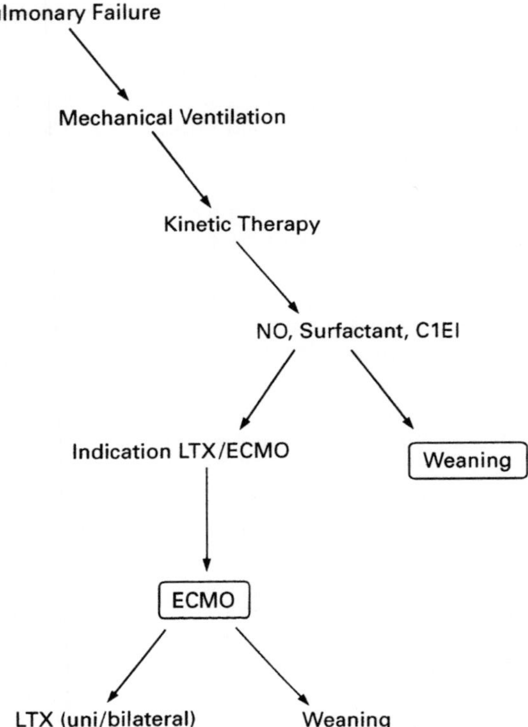

Fig. 1. Therapeutic regime in acute respiratory failure (C1EI = C1-esterase inhibitor, ECMO = extracorporeal membrane oxygenation, LTX = lung transplantation, NO = nitric oxide)

Table 1. Demographic data in seven patients undergoing extracoporeal membrane oxygenation and subsequent lung transplantation for acute respiratory failure (ARDS = adult respiratory distress syndrome, DLTX = double lung transplantation, ECMO = extracoporeal membrane oxygenation, MOV = multiorgan failure, OB = obliterative bronchiolitis, RVF = right ventricular failure, SLTX = single lung transplantation, TEA = thrombendartherectomy)

Patients	Indications	ECMO	TX	Results
32 yrs, female	reperfusion damage (SLTX)	10 days	Re-SLTx	dead (5 months; MOV, OB)
46 yrs, female	acute rejection (SLTX)	1 day	Re-SLTx	alive, 97 months
19 yrs, male	ARDS (trauma)	5 days	DLTX	alive (83 months)
32 yrs, male	ARDS (trauma)	6 days	SLTX	dead (intraop; RVF)
43 yrs, female	ARDS (liver-/kidney-TX)	13 days	SLTX	alive (67 months)
23 yrs, female	unsuccessful pulmonary TEA	2 days	SLTX	dead (13 months; OB)
11 yrs, female	ARDS (trauma)	40 days	adult split lung	alive (33 months)
54 yrs, male	reperfusion damage (DLTX)	5 days	recovered	alive (28 months)

thrombendarterectomy was unsuccessful and due to persistent fixed pulmonary hypertension weaning from cardiopulmonary bypass was only possible by means of ECMO. One patient underwent bilateral sequential lung transplantation in the case of posttraumatic ARDS, while in five patients a single lung procedure (two redo) and in the 11-year-old child bilateral reduced size lung transplantation from an adult donor was performed after a suitable younger donor could not be identified over a period of 4 weeks. The last patient recovered from reperfusion injury after 5 days of ECMO. There was one intraoperative fatality due to intractable right heart failure in combination with pre-existing multiorgan failure. The two late deaths were caused by obliterative bronchiolitis and multiorgan failure 5 resp. 13 months after transplantation. Survival ranges between 2–97 (median 67) months.

Comment

Lung transplantation in acute pulmonary failure including ECMO support represents a complex procedure with acceptable results. Due to the enormous consumption of resources in terms of donor organs, intensive care time and medical cost its application should be restricted to a selected patient group with no concurrent disease. It should also be limited to cardiac surgical centers well experienced in lung transplantation. Indications may represent intractable ARDS following isolated severe thoracic trauma (2) or unspecific pulmonary failure, early graft loss after lung transplantation or persistent pulmonary hypertension after conventional cardiac or pulmonary surgery. Critical issues are the selection of suitable candidates, detection of possible contraindications, the time point of unsuccessful weaning of ECMO and the presumed consent of the individual (3).

Despite the low total number of patients undergoing this combined approach, this series does probably present the largest single center experience worldwide. Approximately two-thirds of the patients will survive this procedure and long-term results seem to be similar to those for "elective" lung transplantation. However, for recommendation of standard criteria with respect to inclusion/exclusion of candidates for this approach and estimation of presumed survival more experience must be gained to re-address the critical issues regarding indications and results.

Summary

A total of eight patients requiring extracorporeal membrane oxygenation for acute pulmonary failure underwent lung transplantation within 1–40 days of bridging. Mean age was 29.4 ± 12.7 years and underlying disease was ARDS (n = 4), reperfusion damage after previous lung transplantation (n = 3), unsuccessful pulmonary thrombendarterectomy (n = 1). One patient underwent bilateral sequential lung transplantation in the case of posttraumatic ARDS, while in five patients a single lung procedure (2 redo) was done. In an 11-year-old child bilateral reduced size lung transplantation was performed. There was one intraoperative fatality caused by intractable right ventricular failure and two late deaths due to obliterative bronchiolitis and multiorgan failure 5 resp. 13 months after transplantation. Survival ranges between 2–97 (median: 67) months. Lung transplantation in acute pulmonary failure including ECMO represents a complex procedure with acceptable results. Due to the enormous consumption of resources in terms of donor organs, intensive care time and medical costs, its application should be restricted to selected patients with no concurrent disease.

References

1. Cooper JD, Trulock EP, Triantafillou AN, Patterson GA, Pohl MS, Deloney PA, Sundaresan RS, Roper CL (1995) Bilateral pneumonectomy (volume reduction) for chronic obstructive pulmonary disease. J Thorac Cardiovasc Surg 109: 106–119.
2. Demertzis S, Haverich A, Ziemer G, Nehrlich M, Müller KM, Wagner TOF, Borst HG (1992) Successful lung transplantation for posttraumatic adult respiratory distress syndrome. J Heart Lung Transpl 11: 1005–1007.
3. Eagan ThM. When is lung transplantation appropriate? 1992 J Heart Lung Transpl 11: 1008.
4. Haverich A, Wagner TOF. Lungen- und Herz-Lungen-Transplantation. In: Cobet R, Gutzeit K, Bock HE (Eds) Klinik der Gegenwart XIII,5 p1-40. Urban und Schwarzenberg, München, Wien, Baltimore 1993.
5. Hosenpud JD, Fiol B, Keck B, Bennett LI (1998) The Registry of the International Society for Heart and Lung Transplantation: Fifteenth Official Report – 1998. J Heart Lung Transplant 17: 656–668.
6. Kallis P, Al-Saady NM, Bennett ED, Treasure T (1993) Early results of intravascular oxygenation. Eur J Cardio-thorac Surg 7: 206–210.
7. Rossaint R, Slama K, Lewandowski K, Streich R, Henin P, Hoppe T, Barth H, Nienhaus M, Weidemann H, Lemmens P, Fuschs J, Falke KJ (1992) Extracorporeal lung assist with heparin coated systems. Int J Art Organs 14: 29–34.

Authors' address:
S.W. Hirt, M.D.
Dep. of Cardiovascular Surgery
Kiel University Hospital
Arnold-Heller-Str. 7
24105 Kiel, Germany

Lung and heart-lung transplantation with direct bronchial artery revascularization

G. Pettersson,[1] M. A. Nørgaard,[1] C. B. Andersen,[3] H. Arendrup,[1] F. Efsen,[4] S. A. Mortensen,[2] P. S. Olsen,[1] U. G. Svendsen,[2]

[1]Department of Thoracic Surgery RT, [2]Department of Medicine B, [3]Department of Pathology, [4]Department of Diagnostic Radiology, Rigshospitalet, National University Hospital, Copenhagen, Denmark

Introduction

The lungs have a dual blood supply, the pulmonary artery low pressure system and the bronchial arteries. The two systems communicate. The bronchial arteries are small arteries that originate in the descending aorta and follow the bronchi far out in the lung parenchyma. Venous drainage is to pulmonary and systemic veins (1, 2), and by precapillary anastomoses into the pulmonary circulation (2).

Single- and double lung transplantations have become therapeutic options for patients with end-stage pulmonary disease (3, 4). In the presuccess era the dominating problem of lung transplantation was airway complications. Ischemia of the central airways was a problem. In the Toronto series single lung transplantation with a "close-to-the-lung" bronchial anastomosis was associated with a low incidence of airway problems, while en-bloc double lung transplantation was still associated with a high incidence of bronchial problems (5). Sequential bilateral lung transplantation was introduced to replace en-bloc double lung transplantation (6). The new technique reduced the incidence of airway complications to a low level (3).

Another option to avoid bronchial ischemia and complications could have been to restore the bronchial artery circulation. Although single lung transplantation with direct revascularization of the bronchial arteries was done experimentally in dogs already in 1950 by Metras (7), most lung transplant surgeons have presumed that direct revascularization is too difficult and too unreliable to be performed clinically. The method used in the first successful lung transplantations, single as well as en-bloc double, to protect the bronchial or tracheal anastomosis was to wrap the anastomosis with omentum (5, 8, 9).

The dependence of the central airways on bronchial artery supply seems clear but the importance of the bronchial arteries to the lungs still remains speculative. There is some evidence that the bronchial artery circulation is of importance to the lung's fluid balance and could reduce posttransplant pulmonary edema (10, 11) and to the lung's resistance and defense against infections (12). It has also been suggested that ischemia could be a factor of importance to the development of bronchiolitis obliterans syndrome (BOS) after transplantation (13).

A number of lung transplant groups (7, 14–18) have tried to develop clinically useful techniques for direct bronchial artery revascularization (BAR) to avoid bronchial complications. An isolated first attempt to revascularize a transplanted lung in a patient was made in 1973 by Haglin et al. (19). Lung transplantation with direct bronchial artery revascularization (BAR) was introduced clinically by Couraud in 1992 (17). Both single and sequential bilateral lung transplantation without BAR are today associated with a low incidence of bronchial problems and only a few groups have adopted and developed the BAR technique (16, 20, 21).

Since the start of the lung transplant program in Denmark in 1992, en-bloc double lung transplantation (DLTX) including BAR has been our preferred method of lung transplantation for most patients and indications. With experience and confidence BAR has, more and more consistently, been attempted also in single lung (SLTX) and heart-lung (HLTX) transplantations.

Surgical technique

Donor operation for lung or heart-lung transplantation with BAR

Any donor with an arterial saturation exceeding 12 kPa on a FiO_2 of 40% is considered a potential lung donor. Imipenem and Methylprednisolon are given to the donor. Cytomegalovirus (CMV) serology mismatch (positive donor to negative recipient) has so far not been accepted. Size matching is based on the calculated total lung capacities of the donor and the recipient and consideration of the recipient's pathology.

The principles of the donor operation are the same as those previously described by Schreinemakers (1990), Couraud (1992), and Daly/Yacoub (1993) (14, 16, 22). The heart and the lungs are removed en-bloc with the trachea, esophagus, and descending aorta. The heart is preserved with St. Thomas solution and the lungs are preserved with modified Euro-Collins solution. A midline sternotomy is used for the donor operation. The lungs are ventilated with 40% O_2 and 5 cm H_2O PEEP during perfusion and at the end allowed to collapse. Organ mobilization and dissection is started at the level of the diaphragm. The organs are mobilized from below and the plane of dissection should be close to the thoracic wall and the spinal column. The pleura is incised longitudinally parallel to the column, on the left side just lateral to the aorta and on the right side 2 cm lateral to the azygos vein. On the right side the dissection is continued at least 3 cm above the azygos vein to avoid injury to the intercostobronchial artery and the right bronchial artery behind the esophagus. Before stapling and dividing the trachea, the lungs are inflated to 50–60 %. If the heart is to be separated from the lung block (as described below) this is preferably done by the recipient surgeon but it may be done at the donor site before, *in situ*, or after removal of the heart-lung bloc.

DLTX recipient operation

High-dose aprotinin is given to the recipient during the operation. The recipient is opened through a midline sternotomy and the left internal mammary artery is prepared. The mammary artery is mobilized close to its origin for maximal length. The pericardium is opened and cannulation sutures are placed. Donor organ arrival is awaited.

The donor organs are inspected and prepared at a side table. If not already done, the heart is separated from the lung block. A 3–5 mm cuff of atrial wall is left with each pair of the pulmonary veins. The main pulmonary artery is divided half way to the bifurcation, ideally 5 mm above the commissures. The esophagus is stripped out by sharp dissection close to the esophageal wall leaving a mediastinal tissue tunnel (Fig. 1). The descending aorta is opened longitudinally in the pleura-covered part of the circumference. The total number of bronchial arteries is most often 1–4 with their orifices in the aorta located in the proximal part of the descending aorta as described below (see : "Surgical bronchial artery anatomy") (Fig. 2). The identification is mainly based on inspection and palpation. Inspection is facilitated by keeping a finger in the esophageal mediastinal tunnel and gentle stretching of the tissue. Probing is done very carefully with a 1 mm probe when necessary, to verify course and branches of an artery. In most cases, the largest artery orifice from the descending aorta is that of the first right segmental artery, the intercostobronchial artery, which goes behind the esophagus to the right lung. The costal branch of this artery is localized and secured by a clip. Revascularization of one major/large bronchial artery may result in complete revascularization, but, if possible, all identified bronchial arteries are revascularized. Excessive tissue is trimmed away, taking care not to interfere with the bronchial artery circulation. After preparation is completed the lungs are stored in ice-cold Ringer-solution.

The recipient is cannulated. A two-stage atrial cannula is normally used but change to bicaval cannulation may be necessary. Cardiopulmonary bypass is started and the patient cooled to 25°C. The heart is fibrillated and an apical left ventricular vent is introduced. A capacitance reservoir (Polystan A/S Copenhagen) is included in the vent line to facilitate regulation of the vent to reduce the risk of left ventricular distention. It is mandatory that the heart is well drained on both sides or the

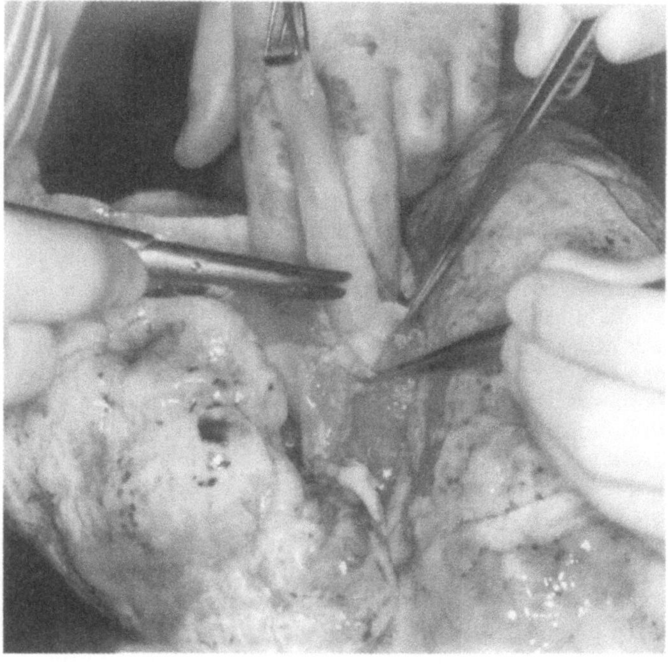

Fig. 1. The esophagus is removed by sharp dissection close to the esophageal wall, leaving a mediastinal tissue tunnel

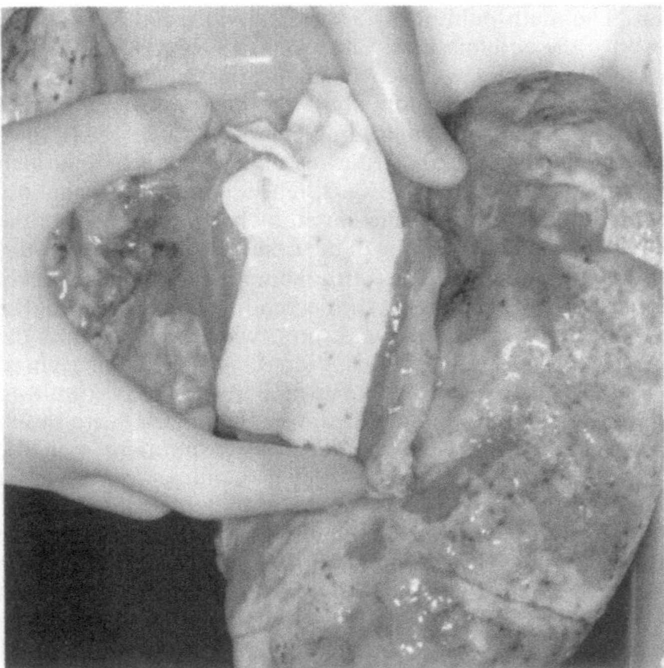

Fig. 2. The opened descending aorta. In the present case the first segmental artery orifice is a double orifice of the intercostobronchial artery and one left bronchial artery

dissection will be less controlled and large amounts of blood have to be handled by the cardiotomy suction. The pleural cavities are opened, inspected, and the phrenic nerves and the left vagal nerve (left recurrent laryngeal nerve) are localized. Removal of the lungs may be accomplished by dividing the main central structures first or last. Dividing the pulmonary arteries, veins, and main bronchi close to the lung first is the easiest and fastest method but is not recommended if the lungs are infected. Contamination of the field by bronchial secretion must be avoided. Hemostasis is well maintained and adhesions are divided by cautery. After removal of the lungs common openings between the pericardium and the pleural cavities are created taking care to avoid injuries to the phrenic nerves and the left recurrent laryngeal nerve. On the left side the pericardial opening is extended superiorly between the phrenic and vagal nerves. The tissue between the left atrium and the pulmonary artery is divided. The pulmonary veins and artery are prepared for the planned anastomoses, considering the conditions dictated by the donor organs. Finally, the main bronchi and carina are dissected close to the bronchial wall. Mediastinal and pleural hemostasis is perfected.

The donor lungs are brought to the operation table. The trachea is opened proximally, bronchial secretion is removed by suction, and the bronchial tree is rinsed with saline. Bronchial secretion is sent for microscopy and culture. The donor trachea is divided one ring above the carina, the level controlled from within the trachea. Peritracheal dissection distal to the level of division is avoided. The lung bloc is introduced into the left pleural cavity and the right lung gently pushed through the pericardial openings and mediastinum behind the heart to the right pleura. The internal mammary artery to bronchial artery anastomosis/es is/are performed first. The left lung is lifted up and hung backwards over the heart thereby exposing the bronchial artery openings in the opened donor descending aorta on top of the heart (Fig. 3). Running 7–0 monofilament suture is used (Fig. 4). Separate sequential anastomoses are preferred when the distance between two bronchial artery openings exceeds a few millimeters. The mammary artery pedicle is anchored to the aortic wall by a few extra sutures. Following removal of the internal mammary artery clamping, successful BAR is immediately evident by bleeding from the donor mediastinal tissue. Before placing the left lung back in the pleura the hemostasis on the backside of the donor organs is checked and significant bleeding is stopped. The mammary artery is left open during the rest of the procedure allowing bronchial artery reperfusion. The remaining anastomoses are performed in the sequence – trachea, left lung veins, right lung veins, and pulmonary artery. The tracheal anastomosis is performed with 4–0 monofilament suture, running in the membranous part and interrupted in the carti-laginous part. The tracheal sutures are tied from in front and backwards forcing any size-discrepancy between donor and recipient trachea to the membranous part. The vascular anastomoses are performed running with 4–0 or 5–0 monofilament sutures depending on tissue quality and vessel size. Rotation, dog-ears, pockets, or stenosis are unacceptable. Available anatomical landmarks are preserved when possible. Ventilation is started and the heart and lungs are deaired. The apical vent is removed and fibrillation stopped. Sinus rhythm often returns spontaneously within a few seconds after removal of the fibrillation. Care must be taken not to disconnect the fibrillation wires accidentally during the rewarming phase. A left atrial catheter for pressure recording is placed through the right upper lung vein. The heart is allowed some filling to ensure transpulmonary flow until weaning from cardiopulmonary bypass. Three drains, one placed posteriorly in each pleura with the tips in the pleural

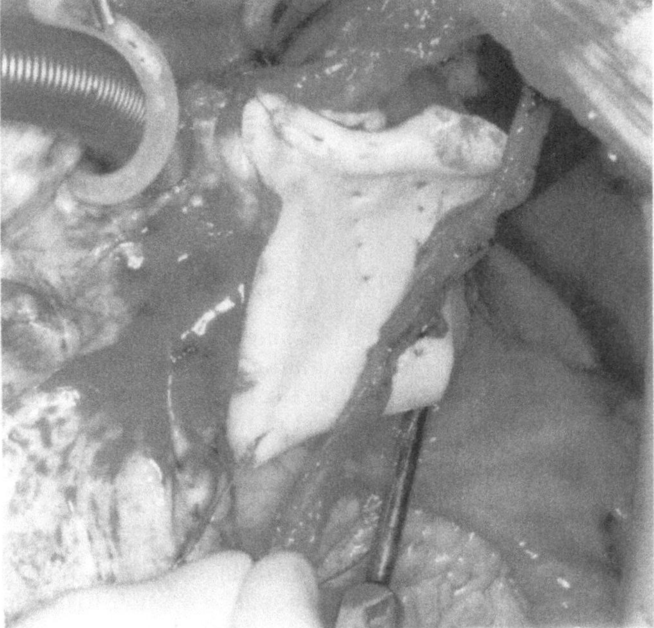

Fig. 3. After introduction of the bloc into the donor, the left lung is lifted up and hung backwards over the heart and the donor descending aorta with the bronchial artery orifices is exposed on top of the heart

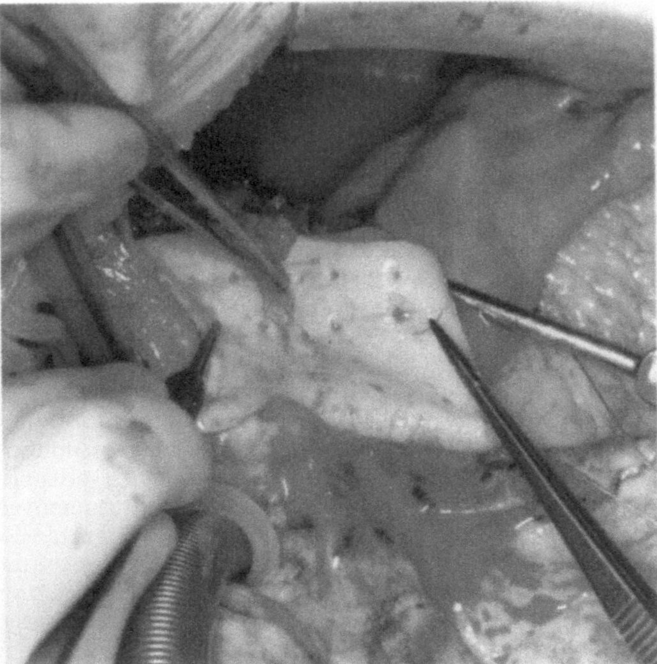

Fig. 4. In this case the mammary artery is only anastomosed to the double orifice. Exposure is excellent

sinuses and one placed retrosternally, are introduced through stabwounds in the epigastrium. The tracheal anastomosis is covered by approximation of nearby recipient and donor peritracheal tissue. Rewarming is completed and the patient weaned from cardiopulmonary bypass, decannulated, and protamine is given. Left atrial pressure above 10 mmHg is avoided. Bronchoscopy is performed for inspection of the anastomosis and clearance of the bronchial tree from blood and secretion.

HLTX recipient operation

The technique of BAR in heart lung transplantation is identical to that described for en-bloc double lung transplantation. The mammary artery to bronchial artery anastomosis/es is/are performed as the first anastomosis/es as in DLTX. Early bronchial reperfusion is allowed. The rest of the procedure is a standard HLTX operation.

SLTX recipient operation

After removal of the heart and bronchial artery identification the lung bloc is divided. In at least 50 % of the cases it should be possible to divide the bloc in such a way that bronchial artery revascularization of both lungs is possible. In SLTX the mammary to bronchial artery anastomosis/es is/are performed last. At this stage backbleeding is observed from the brochial artery orifice(s) verifying that it is a bronchial artery. The donor bronchus is divided in a standard way close to the lung but more of the peribronchial and mediastinal tissue is left with the lung in order to not disturb the bronchial artery circulation.

Postoperative management

The patients are extubated early and aggressive physiotherapy, including CPAP, is started. If problems with bronchial secretion occur or if prolonged ventilatory support is required, the threshold to give the patient a tracheostomy is low. Pleural drains are kept for 3–7 days and sometimes longer. Exudation to the pleural cavities may continue for weeks and may result in progressive hypovolemia. Kidney function may be compromised in the early postoperative period while close monitoring of cyclosporine levels, diuresis, body weight, and fluid balance is important.

Early immunosuppression therapy includes antithymocyte globulin induction 1–5 days (r-ATG, Merieux), methylprednisolone (Solu-Medrol, Upjohn), and azathioprin (Imurel, Glaxo-Wellcome). Maintenance immunosuppression consists of cyclosporine (Sandimmune, Sandoz, from day 1–5), azathioprin, and prednisolone (Prednisolone, Nycomed DAK). Cyclosporine is not started until the patient is circulatory stabile and diuresis is good. Acute rejection is treated with 1 g methylprednisolone daily for 3 days followed by a course of prednisolone 0.5–1 mg/kg/day as starting dose and tapered during 14 days down to the maintenance dose 0.1 mg/kg/day.

Perioperative prophylaxis with ceftriaxon (Rocephalin, Roche) and fusidin (Fucidin, Leo) is given the first 2–5 days. Aciclovir (Zovirax, Glaxo Wellcome) is given for 3 months. Ganciclovir (Cymevene, Roche) is given prophylactically to CMV positive recipients for 2–3 weeks after treatment of acute rejections. Starting after 3–4 weeks, trimethoprim-sulfomethoxazole (Sulfotrim, GEA) is given twice a week.

Bronchoscopy is used liberally when indicated to clear airway secretion and together with bronchoalveolar lavage (BAL) and transbronchial biopsies (TBB) in the diagnosis of infection and rejection.

Lung function (FVC and FEV_1) is monitored daily using a microspirometer.

Patients and methods

Between January 1992 and January 1995, 48 first time DLTX, 9 of 17 HLTX, and 5 of 9 SLTX with BAR have been performed in our department. The DLTX patients suffered from emphysema due to $\alpha - 1$-antitrypsin deficiency (n = 32), chronic obstructive pulmonary disease (n = 11), cystic fibrosis (n = 3), and primary pulmonary hypertension (n = 2). The HLTX patients suffered from Eisenmenger syndrome (n = 7), primary pulmonary hypertension (n = 1), and COLD and cardiomyopathy (n = 1). The SLTX patients suffered from lung fibrosis (n = 2), COLD (n = 2), and emphysema (n = 2).

Bronchoscopy with TBB and BAL is repeated routinely every second week during the first 2 months, and thereafter at 3, 6, 12, 18, and 24 months. After 24 months,

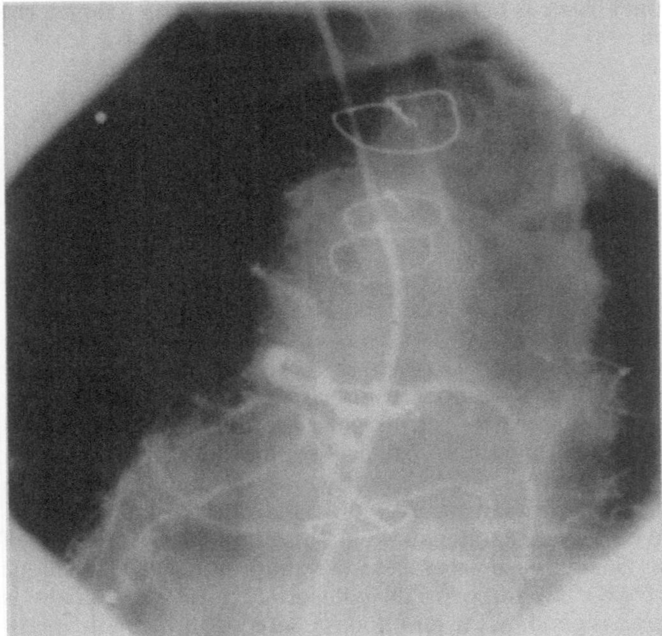

Fig. 5. Postoperative mammary-bronchial arteriography demonstrating complete BAR

bronchoscopy is performed once a year. The international working group formulation criteria (ISHLT) were used for the morphologic evaluation.

Standard complete spirometry is performed regularly.

Arteriographic assessment of LIMA patency and bronchial artery perfusion is routinely performed within 6 weeks postoperatively using Seldinger technique. BAR is considered *successful BAR* if any bronhial artery branch(es) is/are visualized. Successful BAR is classified as *complete BAR* (Fig. 5) if bronchial artery branches for all lung lobes are found, and *incomplete BAR* (subgraded as bilateral, hemilateral, or poor) if visible bronchial artery supply to one or more lobes is/are missing. BAR is classified as *failed BAR* if no bronchial arteries are visualized (23).

Follow-up is complete.

Surgical bronchial artery anatomy and BAR

The bronchial arteries are to be looked for in the proximal part of the descending aorta. An orifice larger than the other, immediately attracting attention, usually includes a bronchial artery. Most often this artery is an intercostobronchial artery found next to the ostium of the first right segmental artery. The intercostobronchial artery branches into an intercostal artery and a right bronchial artery within 1–2 cm from the aorta. Proximal and medial to this artery is sometimes found a subcarinal artery. The subcarinal artery is named by its course, directly towards the subcarinal region. This artery could in reality be the most important right bronchial artery or even a bronchial artery trunk supplying both the right and the left lung. The arteriographically most prominent bronchial artery was a bronchial artery trunk in more than 50% of the cases. A separate right bronchial artery, having its course in front of the esophagus could have its orifice in the area between the subcarinal artery and the first right segmental artery. The left bronchial arteries are most variable in location, number and size. Usually there are 1–3 separate left bronchial arteries. Our ambition has been to revascularize all identified bronchial arteries, but selecting only the largest for revascularization still has a good chance of resulting in complete BAR since this artery is often a bronchial artery trunk.

There is a learning process involved in the surgical identification as well as in the performance of the revascularization. The number of arteries identified and revascularized per case increased with experience. Contributing to this change was improved exposure and introduction of sequential mammary anastomoses. In the 48 DLTX cases, 101 bronchial arteries were identified, of which 89 were revascularized. Thirtythree patients had revascularization of more than one artery, in 13, two or more bronchial artery orifices were covered by a common mammary artery cuff, and in 20, sequential anastomoses were made. Failed identification was the probable cause of failed BAR in one patient. Injury to the intercostobronchial artery during organ harvesting and preparation has occurred three times. In one case BAR was still attempted and incomplete poor BAR achieved, while in the second case (HLTX) the damaged artery was excluded from BAR. In the third case a bronchial artery was perforated with the probe, but the artery was successfully repaired.

Perioperative course and complications

The operation lasted between 2.5 and 8 h. The extra time required for organ procurement, bronchial artery identification, and revascularization is estimated to be 20–45 min. Early bronchial artery reperfusion following the completion of the mammary artery to bronchial artery anastomoses reduced the time of ischemia by 1 h. The heart was kept fibrillating (DLTX) for 2–4 h, corresponding to most of the cardiopulmonary bypass time. Cardiac function was immediately normal in all but one patient (due to coronary artery thrombosis).

All SLTXs were performed without cardiopulmonary bypass.

Five patients, all DLTX, have been reoperated because of bleeding, The mammary anastomosis was the major source of bleeding and required additional hemostatic sutures in three. In one of these patients immediate mammary arteriography showed failed BAR, with occluded anastomoses but an open mammary artery. The mammary anastomoses were redone with a second reoperation through a left-sided thoracotomy. The end result was successful complete BAR (Fig. 6).

Survival

There were no operative deaths. Thirty-day mortality was for DLTX 2.1%, HLTX 0, and SLTX 20% (1 patient). One-year survival was 83% (Kaplan-Meier), 87%, and

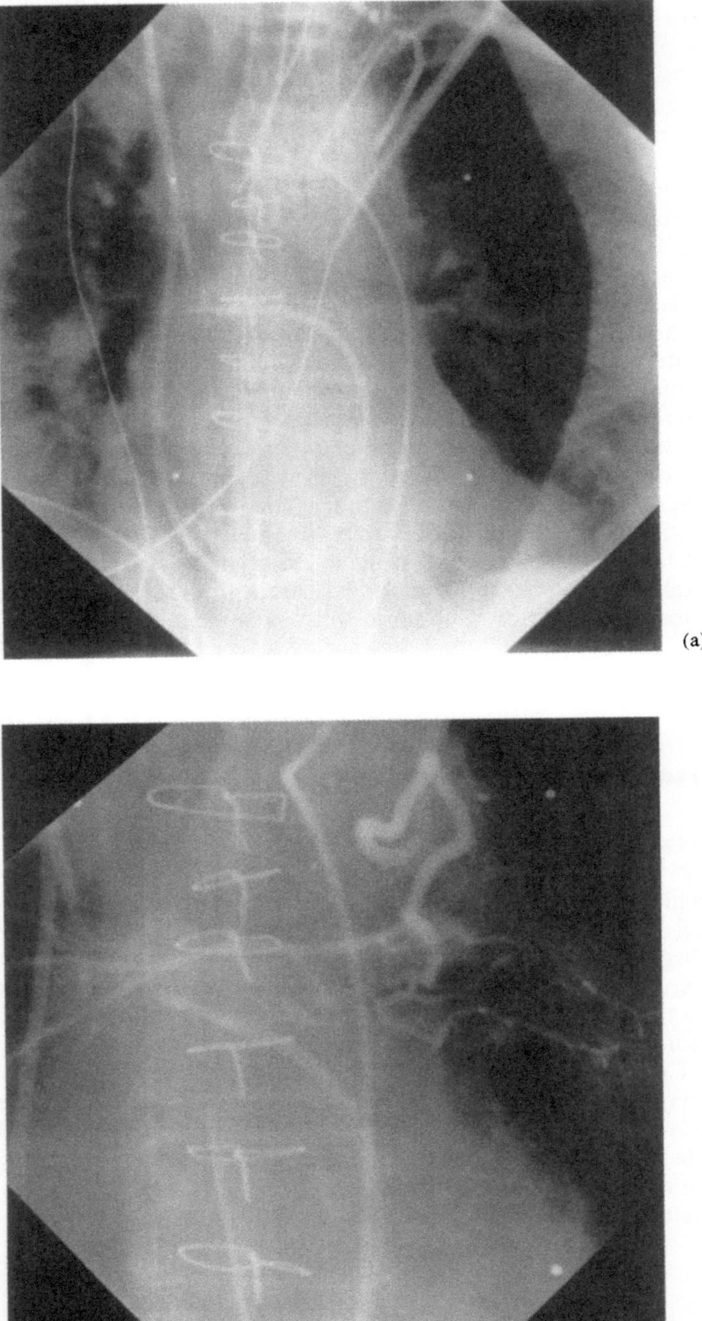

Fig. 6. Failed revascularization verified by mammary-bronchial arteriography immediately after the patient had been reoperated for bleeding from the mammary anastomosis (**a**). The patient was taken back to the operating room and again reoperated through a left thoracotomy and the mammary to bronchial artery anastomoses were redone. The end result was successful complete BAR (**b**)

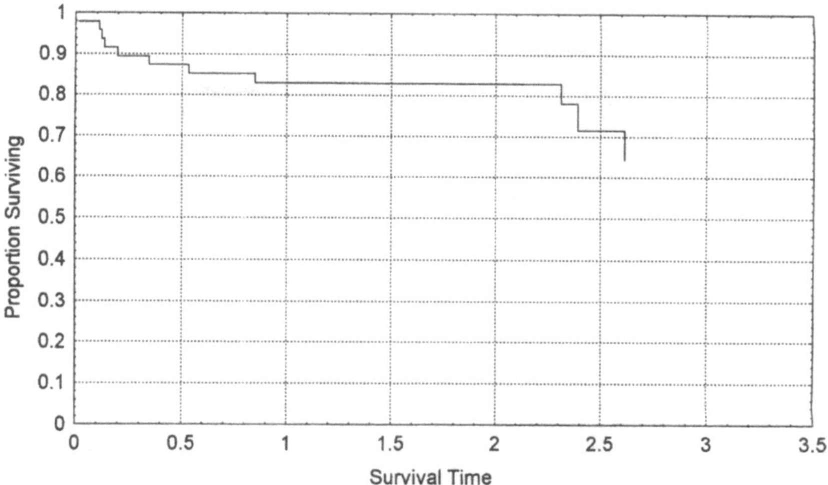

Fig. 7. The proportion of surviving DLTX patients (Kaplan-Meier-plot). The proportion surviving patients versus post-Tx days is shown on the ordinate. The N expresses the number of patients to a certain observation time. One- and 2-year overall survival was 83% and 3-year survival was 62%. (The number of HLTX and SLTX patients is too small to present in survival curves.)

80%, respectively. DLTX survival using Kaplan-Meier technique is found in Fig. 7. Twelve DLTX, 1 HLTX, and 1 SLTX patients have died.

Causes of death after DLTX were: Cerebral infarction after 1 week, pneumonia and lung bleeding after 1.5 months, colon perforation and multi organ failure after 1.5 months, hemorrhagic pancreatitis after 1.5 months, suicide after 2.5 months, lymphoproliferative disease and multi-organ failure after 3.5 months, recurrent rejections and pneumonia after 4 months, BOS and gastrointestinal cytomegalovirus (CMV) infection after 6.5 months, recurrent pneumonias and severe osteoporosis after 10 months, pneumonia after 28 months, recurrent hemorrhagic pancreatitis after 31 months, and BOS after 32 months (retransplanted after 22 months with a right-sided single lung but died 10 months following the retransplantation).

The HLTX patient died from multiorgan failure after 1 month. Contributing to the outcome was a retroperitoneal bleeding from the femoral artery after arteriography.

The SLTX patient was a patient with pulmonary hypertension who died 7 days postoperatively because of acute ventilation perfusion mismatch and severe hypoxia.

Tracheal and bronchial healing

In 43 DLTX patients, normal tracheal healing and a healthy distal bronchial mucosa were observed. Arteriography documented successful BAR in 39 of these, complete in 26, and incomplete in 13. Arteriography was not performed in 4 patients due to early complications and death. Mucosal necrosis (Fig. 8) appeared early postoperatively in the main bronchi of three patients, one died after 6 weeks of pneumonia and lung

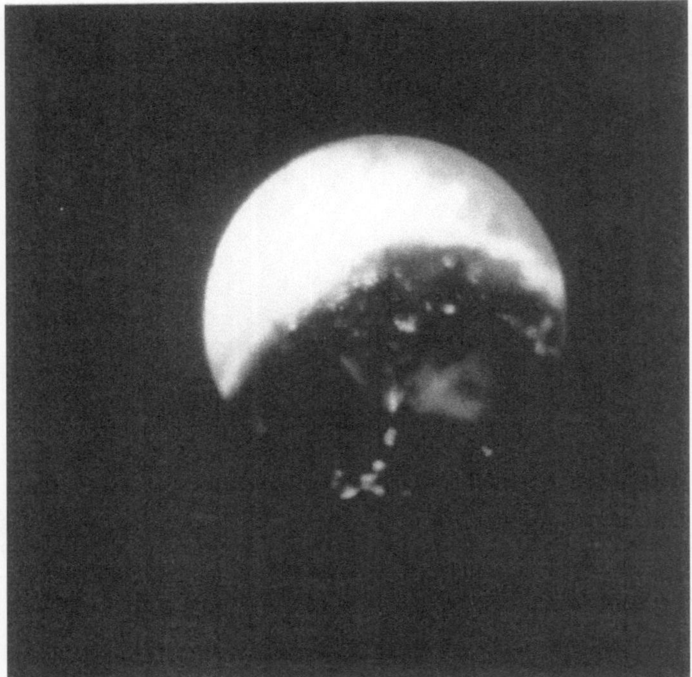

Fig. 8. Necrosis of the bronchial mucosa in a patient with failed BAR

bleeding while the other two survived but developed stenosis of the left main bronchus, eventually requiring left-sided pneumonectomy in both cases. In two patients
local growth of *Aspergillus* distal to the anastomosis required laser evaporation. Both
patients have developed some chondromalacia causing moderate obstruction of the
treated bronchus.

Bronchial healing was normal in all HLTX patients except one who developed an
ulcer in the left main bronchus that healed without sequelae. This patient had
a successful incomplete BAR. There were no bronchial healing problems after SLTX.

Arteriographic results

Arteriography has been performed in 53 patients, 43/48 DLTX, 6/9 HLTX, and 4/6
SLTX. Successful BAR was documented by arteriography in 51 patients and failed
BAR in 2 patients (both DLTX).

BAR in DLTX was complete in 26 (in 1 after reoperation), incomplete in 15
(bilateral in 12, hemilateral in 2, and poor in 1), and failed in two patients.

BAR in HLTX was complete in 3 and incomplete in 3 (bilateral in 1 and hemilateral
in 2). BAR in SLTX was complete in all 4.

Bronchial healing was normal in 9 of the 10 patients who were not examined with
arteriography. In the 10th patient (DLTX) BAR was on clinical findings considered as

failed BAR. The possibility of failed BAR in the 3 HLTX and 2 SLTX patients not examined by arteriography cannot be excluded based on the finding of normal airway healing.

Infections

DLTX

By mistake, there was one CMV mismatch. Twenty-one patients have been treated with a course of ganciclovir (5 mg/kg/day for 2–3 weeks, Cymevene, Roche) on clinical indication. In 4 of these patients evidence of CMV was not demonstrated. Seven patients had 2 or 3 courses of ganciclovir treatment. No patients are believed to have died of CMV infections, although gastrointestinal CMV caused symptoms and nutritional problems during a prolonged period in one patient who died early (6.5 months) from bronchiolitis obliterans syndrome (BOS).

In 11 patients, colonization with *Aspergillus fumigatus* was observed and actively treated. Excluding the two patients discussed above, anastomotic healing was normal. In five patients, airway colonization with *Candica albicans* was observed, but no treatment has been given. In two patients, infection with *Pneumocystis carinii* was diagnosed and treated.

Bacterial infections in the transplanted lungs requiring treatment were observed in 33 patients. *Staphylococcus aureus, Enterobacteriacea*, and *Pseudomonas* species were the most common bacteria. In 8 patients, *Legionella pneumophilia* was observed in the BAL and treated.

HLTX

Four patients have been treated with a course of ganciclovir on clinical indication. In three of these patients evidence of CMV was not demonstrated. Three patients had 2 courses of ganciclovir treatment. No sequelae to CMV infection have been found.

No patients have been infected by *Aspergillus fumigatus.*

Bacterial infection in the transplanted lungs, by *Legionella pneumophilia* was treated in one patient.

In this group there has not been any severe infections nor mortality related to infection.

SLTX

Four patients have been treated with a course of ganciclovir on clinical indication. In three of these patients evidence of CMV was not demonstrated. No sequelae to CMV infection has been found.

No patients have been infected by *Aspergillus fumigatus.*

Bacterial infection in the transplanted lung by *Klebsiella* and *Lactobacillus* species was treated in one patient.

In this group there has not been any severe infections nor mortality related to infection.

Lymphoproliferative disease

Three DLTX patients developed post-transplant Ebstein-Barr related lympho-proliferative disease, one after 2 months (in the liver and bone marrow), one after 8 months (in the lungs), and one after 20 months (in the lungs). The first patient died two months after the diagnosis. In the last two patients the lung lymphomas regressed after lowering the immunosuppression and both patients are alive but have developed BOS.

Lung function

The mean FEV_1 in percent of predicted normal FEV_1 is shown in Fig. 9.

Since the groups (DLTX, HLTX, SLTX) are not very large, standard deviation is quite high (at 6 months standard deviations for DLTX/HLTX/SLTX are respectively 23/33/9, at 12 months 27/25/18 and at 24 months 34/32/21).

BOS

Twelve months after DLTX, 7 of 30 patients (23%) had developed BOS, defined as an irreversible loss of FEV_1 of more than 20% of the best value. After 18 months, 7 of 25 (28%), and after 24 months, 6 of 17 (35%) had BOS. In one patient, BOS followed

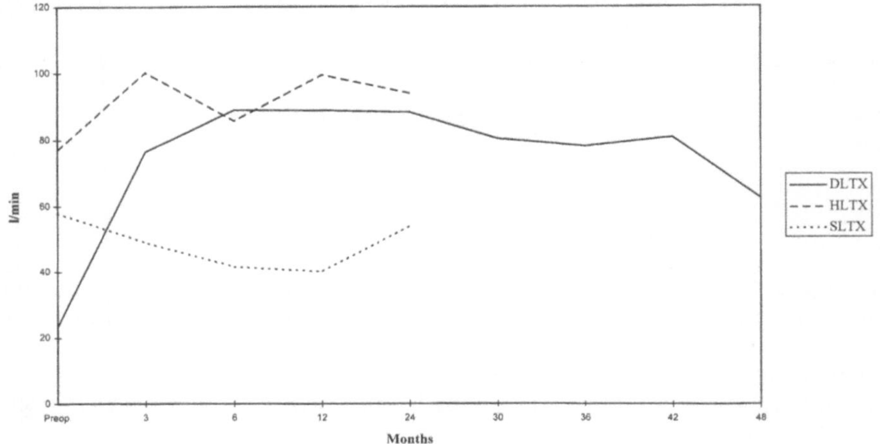

Fig. 9. The FEV_1 in % of the predicted value versus time in months after DLTX, HLTX and SLTX

poor response to treatment of acute rejection, while the other patients had a steady deterioration of lung function over months. The two patients with lymphoproliferative disease in the lungs treated with decreased immunosuppression both developed BOS after 12 and 24 months, respectively.

One HLTX patient has developed BOS after 36 months. FEV_1 has fallen from 103% to 80% of predicted normal.

One SLTX patient has developed BOS after 12 months. FEV_1 has fallen from 52% to 25% of predicted normal after 24 months.

Social status

In January 1996, 36 DLTX, 8 HLTX and 5 SLTX with BAR patients were alive 6–43 months after the transplantation. All patients who had a job before the transplantation returned to work, but no patient unemployed before the transplantation managed to get a job afterwards.

Of the 36 DLTX patients, 11 have returned to work, one is studying and 24 are on early retirement pension.

Of the eight HLTX patients, three have returned to work, one is studying and four are on early retirement pension

Of the five SLTX patients, one is working part time while four are on early retirement pension.

General discussion

The presented method of BAR has proven to be reliable and safe, in DLTX, HLTX, or SLTX. The internal mammary artery is an excellent conduit. The advantage of this conduit compared to vein graft used by Couraud (17), is the prospect of long term patency.

Organ procurement, preparation, and bronchial artery identification are critically important steps, as well as the performance of the mammary to bronchial artery anastomoses. Injuries to the bronchial arteries may occur, and has occurred, during harvesting and preparation. The probe must be used gently. With the present technique, the mammary artery to bronchial artery anastomoses are performed with excellent exposure and donor organ ischemic time is shortened by early bronchial artery reperfusion. The technique of sequential mammary anastomoses has improved BAR further and has reduced the risk of bleeding. With a BAR success rate of 95% en-bloc DLTX with BAR is a viable alternative to sequential bilateral lung transplantation. En-bloc DLTX without BAR should not be performed. Failed BAR in DLTX was associated with severe bronchial problems in two patients and death in one (failed BAR was not arteriographically verified in the last patient). If BAR is to be performed in HLTX and SLTX safety is extra important since BAR in these cases is performed not only to promote airway healing but primarily because of the presumed benefit for the lung(s). It should be underlined that our DLTX series is a consecutive series in which the best possible BAR was attempted in all cases and includes our learning experiences. If failed BAR is suspected, this may be verified by an immediate mammary arteriography. If it is an en-bloc DLTX, the patient should be reoperated through a leftsided thoracotomy and BAR reestablished.

A secondary observation form the DLTX experience is that heart fibrillation at 25°C offers excellent myocardial protection.

Now that we have proven BAR to be possible and safe, we have to prove that it is beneficial for the lungs. Although the bronchial arteries follow the bronchial tree deep into the lungs and it is logical to assume that they are there for a good reason, we still need evidence. Consequently, we are working on a research program to study the bronchial artery circulation and its possible importance to outcome after lung transplantation. Early results after lung transplantation without BAR – single lung as well as sequential bilateral lung – are so good today that it may be argued that BAR is unnecessary and of no proven benefit (24). At the same time, however, we have to remember that long-term results after lung transplantation are still not impressive. The demonstrated safety and good early results requires that the impact of BAR on long-term results after lung transplantation is tested in larger series. To compare clinical outcome after lung transplantation with and without BAR, multicenter cooperation is necessary since no center alone has a sufficiently large number of patients.

Based on the presumption that lungs transplanted with BAR are more resistant against infections, we have not been concerned about steroids in the early postoperative period and we have used an immunosuppressive protocol identical for hearts and lungs. Bacterial infection has been a limited problem. The CMV problem has not been less nor worse than what we have experienced in the heart transplant patients and management has been the same. CMV reactivation as early as 10 days postoperatively has been observed, but only CMV disease, including pneumonia, has been treated. *Aspergillus* and *candida* infections have been observed but have, in all cases, been self-limiting or possible to treat. Obstructing *Aspergillus* growth was in one case related to incomplete poor BAR. Two patients with a previous history of pancreatitis died from hemorrhagic pancreatitis, one early and one late after the transplantation. The cause of death was non-pulmonary in 7 out of 14 lethal cases. Five of these seven patients were stigmatized by steroid medication. As a consequence of the excellent results early in the series (20), the normal acceptance criteria were violated in these cases. We are, however, impressed by the fact that the majority of the patients who have had a complicated course with multi-organ failure have maintained good lung function until death.

Successful BAR resulted in good anastomotic and bronchial healing. When comparing DLTX patients with complete and incomplete BAR, no differences in the clinical outcome are observed. When making this comparison, the critical criteria used to grade BAR as complete must be remembered. Twelve of the 15 patients with incomplete BAR still had a bilateral BAR, only two had a hemilateral, and only one a poor BAR. Successful incomplete bilateral BAR is still good revascularization, and in most cases is probably not associated with any ischemia. Ischemia is probable only with incomplete hemilateral or poor BAR. Other investigators who have performed lung transplantation with BAR have not graded their success. There are two reasons to grade the BAR success; one is to stimulate the surgeon to do a perfect job and the other to allow detailed studies of the clinical importance of revascularization and ischemia, general or local, to the outcome after lung transplantation. It is not enough to compare successful and failed BAR since failed BAR is associated with bronchial complications determining the course. Since BAR in HLTX and SLTX has been introduced more recently, no comparisons between patients with and without BAR have been made yet.

We hope that the reestablished bronchial artery perfusion in the transplanted lungs will reduce the incidence of BOS. This hope is based on the presumption that many factors including ischemia, infections, rejections, and lymphoproliferative disease all may contribute to development of BOS. The present material will, as it grows and follow-up time becomes longer, provide new information about the significance of ischemia to the development of BOS. Our number of long-term survivors is still too small to evaluate the effect on BOS but the figures indicate that BAR does not abolish the BOS problem. Our incidence of BOS seems to be in the same range as that reported by others. A few of the patients regarded as having BOS according to the present definition still have a good function ($\geqslant 50\%$ of predicted normal). Pathoanatomical evidence of obliterative bronchiolitis was not found in all patients with BOS. On the other hand, the distal transbronchial biopsies contain little bronchial tissue.

The majority of the living patients have excellent lung function and are well rehabilitated.

Conclusion

BAR can be performed safely and reliably with any type of lung transplantation, single lung, en-bloc double lung, and heart-lung. The internal mammary artery is an excellent conduit for BAR. En-bloc double lung transplantation with BAR is a viable alternative to sequential bilateral lung transplantation.

The early clinical outcome after lung transplantation with BAR is good and still promising. Larger series and longer follow-up will show whether successful BAR can improve the, still questionable, long-term prognosis after lung and heart-lung transplantation.

Abstract

Background: The lungs have a dual blood supply but most lung transplant surgeons reestablish only the pulmonary artery circulation and neglect the bronchial arteries. Lung transplantation including direct bronchial artery revascularization (BAR) was first done experimentally in the 1940s by Metras but was not introduced clinically until in the 1990s by Couraud et al. BAR has in small series produced promising results.

Methods: In Copenhagen primary en-bloc double lung transplantation (DLTX) with BAR using the left mammary artery as conduit has been the most common method of lung transplantation performed in 48 patients from June 1992 to January 1996. After introduction of the bloc into the recipient the mammary to bronchial artery anastomosis/-es is/are performed as the first anastomosis/-es allowing perfect exposure and early reperfusion. An identical technique of BAR has been used in 9 heart-lung transplantations (HLTX) and an adjusted technique has been applied in 5 single lung transplantations (SLTX). The arteriographic results and clinical outcome have been studied.

Results: Arteriography performed in 43 DLTX patients demonstrated successful BAR in 41, complete in 26 and incomplete in 15, and failed BAR in 2. Successful BAR was arteriographically verified also in 6 of 6 examined heart-lung and in 4 of 4 examined single lung transplantations. This means a total arteriographic BAR success rate of 96% (51 out of 53 examined patients). Bronchial healing was normal in 52, disturbed in 3 (2 DLTX, 1 HLTX), and complicated in 3 (DLTX). Five patients, all DLTX, were reoperated for bleeding. Bronchial healing problems were associated with incomplete or failed BAR. Thirty-day and 1-year survival (Kaplan-Meier) for transplantations including BAR were for DLTX 97%/83%, HLTX 100%/87%, and SLTX 80%/80%.

Conclusions: BAR can be performed safely and reliably with any type of lung transplantation, single lung, double lung, and heart-lung. The internal mammary artery is an excellent conduit for BAR. Early results are good and follow-up will show if long-term results will be improved by BAR. En-bloc double lung transplantation with BAR is a viable alternative to sequential bilateral lung transplantation.

References

1. Liebow AA (1965) Patterns of origin and distribution of the major bronchial arteries in man. Am J Anat 117: 19
2. Wagenvoort CA, Wagenvoort N (1967) Arterial anastomoses, bronchopulmonary arteries, and pulmobronchial arteries in perinatal lungs. Lab Invest 16: 13–24
3. Cooper JD (1990) The evolution of techniques and indications for lung transplantation. Ann Surg 212: 249–255
4. Khaghani A et al. (1991) Medium-term results of combined heart and lung transplantation for emphysema. J Heart Lung Transplant 10: 15–21
5. Patterson GA, Todd TR, Cooper JD, Pearson FG, Winton TL, Maurer J (1990) Airway complications after double lung transplantation. Toronto Lung Transplant Group. J Thorac Cardiovasc Surg 99: 14–20
6. Pasque MK, Cooper JD, Kaiser LR, Haydock DA, Triantafillou A, Trulock EP (1990) Improved technique for bilateral lung transplantation: rationale and initial clinical experience. Ann Thorac Surg 49: 785–791
7. Metras H (1950) Note preliminaire sur la greffe totale du poumon chez le chien. C R Acid Sci (Paris) 231: 1176–1178
8. Lima O, Goldberg M, Peters WJ, Ayabe H, Townsend E, Cooper JD (1982) Bronchial omentopexy in canine lung transplantation. J Thorac Cardiovasc Surg 83: 418–421
9. The Toronto Lung Transplant Group (1988) Experience with single-lung transplantation for pulmonary fibrosis. JAMA 259: 2258–2262
10. Pearse DB, Wagner EM (1994) Role of the bronchial circulation in ischemia-reperfusion lung injury. J Appl Physiol 76: 259–265
11. Pearse DB, Wagner EM, Sylvester JT (1993) Edema clearance in isolated sheep lungs. J Appl Physiol 74: 126–132
12. Charan NB, Turk GM, Dhand R (1985) The role of bronchial circulation in lung abscess. Am Rev Respir Dis 131: 121–124
13. Yousem SA, Dauber JH, Griffith BP (1990) Bronchial cartilage alterations in lung transplantation. Chest 98: 1121–1124
14. Schreinemakers HH et al. (1990) Direct revascularization of bronchial arteries for lung transplantation: an anatomical study [see comments]. Ann Thorac Surg 49: 44–53
15. Laks H et al. (1991) New technique of vascularization of the trachea and bronchus for lung transplantation. J Heart Lung Transplant 10: 280–287
16. Daly RC, Tadjkarimi S, Khaghani A, Banner NR, Yacoub MH (1993) Successful double-lung transplantation with direct bronchial artery revascularization [see comments]. Ann Thorac Surg 56: 885–892
17. Couraud L et al. (1992) Bronchial revascularization in double-lung transplantation: a series of 8 patients. Bordeaux Lung and Heart-Lung Transplant Group [see comments]. Ann Thorac Surg 53: 88–94
18. Pettersson G et al. (1996) Surgical Techniques for Én-bloc Double Lung Transplantation and Direct Bronchial Artery Revascularization.. Submitted for publication

19. Haglin JJ, Ruiz E, Baker RC et al.; Wildevur C, editors. Morphology in lung transplantation. Basel, Switzerland: S. Karger, 1973; Histologic studies of human lung allotransplantation. p. 13–22
20. Pettersson G et al. (1994) Early experience of double-lung transplantation with bronchial artery revascularization using mammary artery. Eur J Cardiothorac Surg 8: 520–524
21. Daly RC, McGregor CG (1994) Routine immediate direct bronchial artery revascularization for single-lung transplantation. Ann Thorac Surg 57: 1446–1452
22. Couraud L et al. (1992) Lung transplantation with bronchial revascularisation. Surgical anatomy, operative technique and early results. Eur J Cardiothorac Surg 6: 490–495
23. Nørgaard MA, Efsen F, Olsen P, Svendsen UG, Pettersson G (1996) Surgical and Arteriographic Results of Bronchial Artery Revascularization in Lung- and Heart-Lung Transplantation. Submitted for publication
24. Patterson GA (1993) Airway revascularization: is it necessary? [editorial; comment]. Ann Thorac Surg 56: 807–808

Authors' address:
Gösta Pettersson, M.D., Ph.D.
Department of Cardio-Thoracic Surgery
The National University Hospital (Rigshospitalet)
Blegdamsvej 9
2100 Copenhagen, Denmark

MIX
Papier aus verantwortungsvollen Quellen
Paper from responsible sources
FSC® C105338

If you have any concerns about our products,
you can contact us on
ProductSafety@springernature.com

In case Publisher is established outside the EU,
the EU authorized representative is:
Springer Nature Customer Service Center GmbH
Europaplatz 3, 69115 Heidelberg, Germany

Printed by Libri Plureos GmbH
in Hamburg, Germany